This new edition of
You CAN Do Something About AIDS
is made possible through the generosity and support
of the following companies:

The American Booksellers Association
Canadian Pacific Forest Products, Limited
Ingram Book Company
BPMC: Offset Paperback Manufacturers, Inc.
Alyson Publications, Inc.

Other sponsors:
The Book-of-the-Month Club • Bantam Doubleday Dell
Random House, Inc. • Harper & Row, Publishers
Association of American Publishers
Boise Cascade Corp. • Simon & Schuster • Waldenbooks
Workman Publishing Company • Publishers Weekly

• **Contributors:**
Houghton Mifflin • Addison Wesley
New American Library/E.P. Dutton/Viking Penguin
McGraw Hill Book Company • Abbeville Press
Avon Books • Little, Brown and Company
Library Journal, School Library Journal
John Wiley & Sons • William Morrow Company
Oxford University Press • Zebra Books/Pinnacle Books
The New Republic • Brooks/Cole, PWS-Kent, and Wadsworth

Southern Christian University Library

You CAN
Do Something
About AIDS

Sasha Alyson, editor

RA
644   You can do something about AIDS   00051282
.A25
Y68
1990

A public service project
of the publishing industry

Copyright © 1988, 1990 by The Stop AIDS Project, Inc., a non-profit corporation. All rights reserved. Published by The Stop AIDS Project, 40 Plympton St., Boston, MA 02118.

Photo credits: p. 7: Mary Ann McQuillan; p. 9: John Kings; p. 13: Jane Rosett; p. 19: Patricia Pingree; p. 31: Don Dickson; p. 39: William Morris Agency; p. 45: The Mayne Studio; p. 49: Diane Wayman; p. 56: Kevin Kerdash; p. 63: © 1987 Warner Bros., Inc.; p. 70: NYU/Philip Gallo photo; p. 87: Amy Fish; p. 90: Hallmark Photographers; p. 92: © Kent Garvey; p. 101: Steve Piersol; p. 107 (l): Dell Richards, (r): Hope Harris; p. 121: © 1988 by Johansen Photography; p. 129 (l): Jasper Jorgensen; p. 133: William Garrett; p. 145: Ron Rutkowski; p. 156: Francesco Scavullo; p. 159: Richard H. Merle; p. 161: Jane Rossett; p. 165: Wallace Ackerman Studio.

First edition: May 1988
Second editon: February, 1990
Library of Congress Catalog Card Number 88-090577

ISBN 0-945972-02-4

You CAN Do Something About AIDS is available in bulk to schools, churches, businesses, AIDS organizations, and other groups at a special low price. For details, see page 181.

Contents

SASHA ALYSON: *Foreword,* 7
JAMES A. MICHENER: *Preface,* 9
ELIZABETH TAYLOR: *Introduction,* 13

1: GETTING STARTED
JAMES CARROLL: *Change starts with our own attitudes,* 19
DR. REED TUCKSON: *You can make my job easier,* 22
SEN. LOWELL WEICKER, JR.: *Write your elected officials,* 25
DR. C. EVERETT KOOP: *Looking to the future,* 28
KEVIN GEORGE: *Support your local AIDS group,* 31
JEFFREY ZASLOW: *Education doesn't happen only in schools,* 34

2: EVERYONE CAN MAKE A DIFFERENCE
GREG LOUGANIS: *Be a buddy,* 39
KATE CAPPS: *Volunteer your time,* 42
JOHN PRESTON: *Little extras that make a difference,* 45
REP. HENRY WAXMAN: *The urgent need for research,* 47
JODY POWELL: *Working with the media,* 49
CLEVE JONES: *The Names Project,* 53
JOHN-MANUEL ANDRIOTE: *Show your appreciation,* 56
CHELSEA PSYCHOTHERAPY ASSOCIATES:
    When a friend has AIDS, 59
WHOOPI GOLDBERG: *Think creatively,* 63

3: AT HOME
ABIGAIL VAN BUREN: *An open letter to parents,* 67
RONALD AND ANN MOGLIA: *Talking to your children,* 70
ELIZABETH WINSHIP: *Talking to your parents about AIDS,* 75
EILEEN DELAMADRID: *Children with AIDS need love, too,* 78
RYAN JAMES: *The Pet Pals Program,* 81

4: IN SCHOOL AND CHURCH
JEFF LAVIN'S CLASS: *What a high school class can do,* 87
STEPHEN R. SROKA: *What teachers can do,* 90

ERIC E. ROFES: *Working with your local school board,* 92

SANDRA L. CARON: *AIDS action on campus,* 95

REP. GEORGE MILLER: *Other ways of educating our children,* 98

ZAL SHERWOOD: *How congregations respond to AIDS,* 101

5: IN THE WORKPLACE

DELL RICHARDS: *When a co-worker has AIDS,* 107

LAWRENCE H. WILLIFORD:
Does your workplace policy cover AIDS? 110

ALAN EMERY: *Taking sensible precautions on the job,* 113

BRYAN LAWTON: *Setting the tone in your company,* 116

BILL OLWELL: *A union approach to AIDS in the workplace,* 118

FATHER WILLIAM J. WOOD, S.J.:
Clergy have a unique role in confronting AIDS, 121

JOE DAVIDSON: *Journalists: Get the story right,* 124

GEORGE APPLEBY: *The special challenge for social workers,* 127

JANE PINSKY AND DONNA RAE RICHARDSON:
What health workers can do, 129

HARVEY FIERSTEIN: *People in the arts
have no end of choices,* 133

6: GOING FURTHER

BEN STROHECKER: *The leadership is you,* 137

RAYMOND L. FLYNN: *What a caring city can do about AIDS,* 141

BILL McBRIDE: *Raising funds for AIDS services,* 145

LAWRENCE DEYTON AND JOHN Y. KILLEN, JR.:
Volunteering for a study, 149

TOM SOLES: *Starting an AIDS hotline,* 152

BEVERLY JOHNSON: *Taking action in
minority communities,* 156

MITCHELL CUTLER: *Starting a buddy program,* 159

MICHAEL CALLEN: *C.R.I.s: A creative approach
to AIDS research,* 161

JAMES L. HOLM: *Taking the next step,* 165

APPENDIX

DIRECTORY OF AIDS-RELATED ORGANIZATIONS, 171

FURTHER READING: THE BEST BOOKS ABOUT AIDS, 175

TELEPHONE LISTINGS FOR LOCAL AND
STATE ORGANIZATIONS, 182

SOME THANK-YOU'S

ALL BOOKS REFLECT the cooperative efforts of many people and companies. With this particular book, for which everything from writing and editing to paper, printing, and distribution has been donated, that is even more true.

In the two years since *You Can Do Something About AIDS* was originally conceived, hundreds of people and companies have freely given time, services, money, and support to make it a reality. The largest monetary contributors are credited on the first page, but there are others without whom it would not have been published.

The original inspiration for the book came from Jeff Seroy of Oxford University Press. Early and helpful encouragement, at a point when many in the industry dismissed the idea as impractical, came from Leonore Fleischer, John Preston, Mario Sartori, and Allan Marshall.

As the project progressed, Congressman Gerry Studds gave generously of his time. His hundreds of phone calls opened many doors that would otherwise have remained closed. Others who made exceptional contributions include Martin Weinkle, Buddenbrooks bookstore, Mark S. Smith, and my assistant, Karen Barber, whose competent help has made a dramatic difference in moving the project along.

Fundraising, not surprisingly, was the toughest aspect of this project. Certain companies and organizations took the lead at critical points; they are the American Booksellers Association, the Book-of-the-Month Club, Harper & Row, Ingram Book

Company, the Bantam Doubleday Dell group, and Offset Paperback Manufacturers.

Many individuals within various publishing houses took the initiative in calling this project to the attention of the appropriate executives. Without their support — and, often, their persistence — the book could never have been published.

Etienne Delessert and Rita Marshall captured the spirit of the project with a beautiful cover design and artwork for both the original book, and the new edition.

In addition to the individuals whose names appear on each chapter, other people helped with editorial planning, writing, and editing. They include Robert Riger, Peter Millis, Wayne Curtis, Sandy MacLeod, Lori Abrams, Bill Misenhimer, Brooks Peters, Tim Westmoreland, Maureen Byrnes, Susan Swift, Kathleen Much, Ann Abrams, Christopher McGahan, Christina Coffin, Ana M. Fores, Robert Dirmeyer, and Steve Carlson.

Many individuals within the publishing and bookselling community helped out in other ways. They include Neal Webb, Tara Masih, Ed McGill, Jay Moench, Michael Kazan, Maureen O'Brien, Renee Vera Cafiero, Dick Gladstone, Rob Shepard, Andy Neilly, Vito Perillo, Parker Ladd, B.J. Stiles, Arnold Dolin and Gary Luke, Michael Carlisle, David Groff, John Allison, Paul Reed, Nancy Bereano, Diane Rennert, Simon Michael Bessie, Faith Hornby Hamlin, Roy Finamore, LeDogg, Carol Seajay, Gregor Jamroski, Ira Silverberg, and Richard Robinson.

Other people donated their time, contacts, information, support, and skills as appropriate. I especially want to thank Alec Gray, Joe Chapple, Michael Connolly, Tom Downey, Steve Rabin, Dr. Michael Samuels, Kevin George, Jim Hill, Stephen Hunt, Larry Kessler, John Hoffman, Ron Holder, Nathan Kolodner, Maureen O'Brien, Elizabeth Mehren, Jane Silver, Phyllis Gurdin and Karen Schlachter, Dan Horowitz, Jeanne Phillips, Jim Babbitt, Kathleen Matthews, and Jane Rosett.

Publicity help came from Annik LaFarge of Random

House, Arlynn Greenbaum at John Wiley & Sons, Jeff Johnson, Marcia Powell, Peter Cassels, Nancy Fish at Abbeville Press, Dennis Rhodes, Colleen Murphy at the Book-of-the-Month Club, and Vince Lardo.

In addition, I know that many people helped this project in ways that have never come to my attention. You know who you are, and your contributions did make a difference.

This chapter, like the other chapters in this book, has something to be learned from it. There were certainly times when it seemed like nothing was going right, but at every stage of its growth, the effort to write, publish and disseminate this book has received surprisingly strong support, often from unexpected quarters. If, after reading it, you feel inspired to undertake a major AIDS-related project, I think you'll be surprised and gratified by the support that materializes for your efforts. And perhaps, like me, you'll find that the wonderful people you meet while doing work like this provide one of its greatest unexpected rewards.

—Sasha Alyson

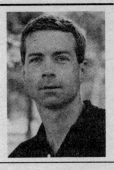

Sasha Alyson

FOREWORD

Sasha Alyson is the president of Alyson Publications in Boston, and coordinator of the project that produced this book.

THIS BOOK IS THE RESULT of a cooperative effort by the publishing community to volunteer its resources in the fight against AIDS. Every step of the way, people in the publishing industry donated the time and services necessary to put this book into your hands. The writing, printing, paper, and publicity work were all contributed.

Never before has the publishing industry united on such a scale to produce a public-service book. But the threat posed by AIDS is so great, and the need for action is so urgent, that nearly every major publishing company has agreed to participate.

The original idea for this book came in 1987, as I talked to other people in publishing about the growing AIDS epidemic. Fashion, entertainment, and other industries had all found a way to help in the fight against AIDS. We asked ourselves: how can the publishing industry do its share?

In June, I decided that a book like this was one thing we could do. I circulated a rough proposal among a few editors and writers I knew, and their responses encouraged me to go ahead. In the year that followed, literally hundreds of people and companies donated freely of their time, services, and money to make this book a reality. Because of those donations, *You CAN*

Do Something About AIDS carries a nominal one-dollar cover price — merely enough to meet the cost of future printings.

Several points should be kept in mind as you read. Most important: *This book does not cover everything you need to know about AIDS*. It has one specific purpose: to offer ideas about concrete action you can take.

It does not discuss AIDS prevention and safe-sex guidelines. Nor does it more than scratch the surface of what you'll want to know if you, or someone you love, has AIDS. Those subjects are crucially important — but the information is readily available elsewhere. The bibliography at the end will guide you to some of the best sources.

Many of the suggestions here are just enough to get you started. Once you find an idea that appeals to you — organizing a fundraiser, for example — you'll probably want further advice. Some chapters list follow-up ideas at the end; you can also ask your local bookseller, librarian, or AIDS organization for suggestions about related material.

You don't need to read *You CAN Do Something About AIDS* front-to-back, and you probably shouldn't. Not every chapter is meant for everyone. Some overlap.

I suggest you start with the first four chapters. They'll give you a sense of things everyone can do, and what this book is about. Then look down the table of contents and see what chapters address your own interests and situation. As you leaf through the book, some chapters will stand out. This book is meant as a springboard to help you and others in your community get involved. You'll soon be amazed by how much you can accomplish.

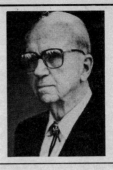

James A. Michener
PREFACE

James Michener, the author of thirty-six books, is one of America's best-known and best-loved authors. His most recent novels are Journey *and* Caribbean.

THREE TIMES DURING MY WORK as a writer I have had to conduct extensive research on plagues, and always I have tried to inject myself into the actual setting of those who were afflicted with the disease and those who were striving to combat it. It has been a mind-shattering experience.

In my early studies on Biblical times I did much work on leprosy, poring over those two dreadful chapters of Leviticus, 13 and 14, in which 116 verses concentrate on this affliction in harrowing detail, including the fearful judgment: "When the plague of leprosy is in a man . . . he shall be defiled; he is unclean; he shall dwell alone; without the camp shall his habitation be."

In writing about Hawaii I chose to live for some time among the lepers on that forlorn site on Molokai, where the afflicted from the other islands were isolated. Death was their only help until the Belgian priest Father Damien sacrificed his own life to assist them.

When writing about the hordes of Americans who crossed the great plains on their way to California and Oregon in the 1840s I was appalled to learn how many died from an inexplicable sweep of cholera through their ranks. Its effect upon travelers alone and untended on the empty prairie must have been pitiful.

As a consequence of focusing on such disasters and, in a sense, living through them personally, I have developed certain conclusions.

1. The onset of any plague is always mysterious, terrifying, and first interpreted as a wrathful visitation of the gods upon sinners.

2. Invariably it evokes frenzied and usually ineffective responses.

3. In time, scientific solutions are discovered, often centering on simple hygiene, but just as often depending on medical discoveries.

4. Each plague ultimately finds its own solution. Even leprosy is now controllable.

5. And in the course of dealing with it, saints of the noblest character evolve, like the men and women of the Old Testament who nursed lepers, like Jesus who cured them, and like Father Damien who gave his life to console them.

My own preoccupation with plagues, and my convictions that one would probably appear in my lifetime, drove me to formulate a sixth rule which I would apply only to myself, but which I do recommend to others: "If a new plague attacks my society I shall try to view it non-hysterically, arrange sensible procedures to comfort the victims, and devote my energies toward the discovery of a cure."

Therefore, when the acquired immune deficiency syndrome (AIDS) struck I could not be surprised, for I knew that throughout history curses as well as blessings appeared cyclically, but I did not foresee that the new plague would be so mysterious, so immune to treatment, and so fatal. Prepared though I was for its coming, in reality it was terrifying.

The time has come for all of us to encourage our society and our government to launch a solid-front attack on AIDS, to disseminate truthful information about it, to provide maximum help to those who have contracted it, and if death becomes inevitable, to make it as gentle and dignified as possible.

I have a special obligation since AIDS has struck so heavily in the artistic community with which I have been associated. It would be shameful for me to castigate in any way the young people who have contracted this disease or in any way ostracize them. They are my brothers and sisters. Children who have automatically inherited the disease are my responsibility. And I must do all in my power to help the afflicted.

AIDS is best seen as merely the latest in a chain of plagues which go back more than three thousand years. It was probably inescapable and will doubtless be duplicated in some unpredictable form within the next two or three centuries. We have reason to hope that we will soon have effective means of combatting it, and that it will not terrorize society as long as leprosy did. Certainly we have more humane ways of responding to it than the hysterical ways outlined in Leviticus and reported in the accounts of previous plagues.

The publishing companies of America are to be applauded for giving the public this sensible, caring, hopeful book. I hope it will be read by millions, for it shows us what we can do to help combat this strange and awesome epidemic.

Southern Christian University Library
1200 Taylor Rd.
Montgomery, AL. 36117

Elizabeth Taylor

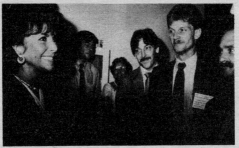

INTRODUCTION

Elizabeth Taylor, shown here talking to a group of people with AIDS who have been lobbying in the U.S. Senate, is the national chairman of the American Foundation for AIDS Research.

THE AIDS CRISIS HAS BROUGHT US face to face with complex medical and social challenges unparalleled in this century. The magnitude of this tragic epidemic is measured not only in the cost of human lives, but also the enormous financial burdens of health care and lost productivity which each and every one of us, as well as future generations, will ultimately bear.

There are two epidemics of AIDS: an epidemic of illness and an epidemic of fear. The costs of the epidemic of fear are immeasurable — the destruction of sane and rational behavior, needless and inhumane discrimination — and, often, the destruction of relationships at a time when they are most needed.

The epidemic of AIDS is also personal. Every day, more and more human beings, most often in the prime of their lives, are told they have AIDS or an AIDS-related condition. Being confronted with the possibility of death presents personal challenges that are truly overwhelming. Few people are able to face these challenges alone. As compassionate people, we must be there to help.

In the face of the severity of the AIDS crisis and its far-reaching consequences, some people feel that the problem is so big there is nothing one person can do that will make a difference, or that someone else or some organization will take care of the problem. Other people, who are more directly affected by AIDS, may feel that they must do something for their own sake or that of their loved ones. There are still others who would like to do something, but aren't sure what is needed.

This book will help provide concrete examples of what *anyone* can do to make a contribution in the fight against AIDS. This book will provide examples of things that can be done in all areas of the AIDS crisis, such as getting informed and educating your children, parents, friends, or acquaintances, writing a letter to your elected officials to let them know how you feel, volunteering for AIDS-related activities, raising money, protecting yourself and others, or changing attitudes. It provides information that can be followed by anyone, including parents, children, teens, members of the clergy, elected officials, students, co-workers, and friends.

William Wordsworth once wrote: "Small service is true service . . . the daisy, by the shadow that it casts, protects the lingering dewdrop from the sun." It's easy to feel that what we can do is too small to make a difference. In reality, many of our actions, no matter how small, may brighten someone's life without our knowledge. And in the long run, all actions will meld and grow into a profound contribution.

You CAN Do Something About AIDS contains many examples of things that everyone can do. One point I would like to stress is that you *express* your concern for the well-being of others. Call to offer help, or just let someone know you are thinking about them, and tell them you love them — send a card or flowers. Keep them informed of positive news. Support them in their decisions. Spend time with them to share their emotions.

This book is meant as a starting point for all citizens to take an active role in defeating AIDS and helping those in need.

The more you participate, the more rewarded you will become. For after all, the privilege of serving others is truly the greatest reward.

1

GETTING STARTED

James Carroll
CHANGE STARTS WITH OUR OWN ATTITUDES

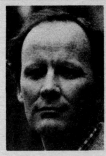

James Carroll is the author of seven novels, the most recent of which is Firebird. *He is married to the novelist Alexandra Marshall. They have two children, Lizzy and Pat, and live in Boston.*

FEAR, ANGER, AND THE URGE to blame — these are among our most common responses to AIDS. Some of our most instinctive attitudes about this disease are negative ones; if we don't admit that and work to understand why it is so, such attitudes can control our decisions in very destructive ways. They can cause a spiritual infection of the moral atmosphere in which we live with each other, and *that* infection will make the urgent tasks of education and prevention of the *physical* disease much more difficult. By admitting our negative attitudes and understanding that they are in some way natural, we can begin to change them.

First, fear. We are right, of course, to be afraid. AIDS is a graphic reminder of the terribly fragile nature of all life on earth. Because it is most commonly transmitted through sexual contact and needle-sharing — activities that are already emotionally loaded — AIDS is doubly fearsome. But the *real* reasons for fearing AIDS are bad enough without adding to them. Runaway fear can exaggerate the threat, making it seem, for example, far easier to catch the disease than it is, and ironically such exaggeration can undermine the reasonableness of our responses, making us all more vulnerable to AIDS than we need to be. The antidote to fear is reliable information. We should know how to check out the inevitable rumors and where to go with our questions. It is to this need that this book is addressed, of course. Its assumption — what we need constantly to remind ourselves of — is that, while AIDS cannot as yet be cured, it *can* be prevented.

But no matter what we do from here on, many people already have the disease and many more are going to get it. And that sure knowledge is what makes us so angry. Because death from AIDS strikes those among us — young, active people — who are most alive, it seems even more outrageous than other deaths. Because it strikes the addicted, to whom life has already been overly cruel, it is especially infuriating. Because it hangs most threateningly over our children as they become sexually mature, it makes us want to strike out.

But at whom? Anger about AIDS is too often directed at those who have been most vulnerable to the disease, as if *they* caused it. Homosexuals are the most common targets of such scapegoating, but now the addicted are becoming the new pariahs of AIDS. Even when we act from good intentions we often dehumanize those who are infected. If we reach out to those most vulnerable to the disease, it is not to "help" the "sick" or the "poor" or "victims" — such words reflect an attitude of patronizing superiority — but because we are all in this together now. There is no superiority and there is no distance; AIDS attacks the immune system of society too. Now no one is immune. Thus those things that have always cut us off from one another — sexism, homophobia, racism, hatred of addicts — have the additional effect now of making this disease more powerful. However understandable the common impulse to blame is, however "human" it is, the fact now is that we indulge it at our common peril.

The climate in which prevention thrives is marked not by blaming, but by caring. It is marked by the frank and open exchange of real information, even information that we once regarded as inappropriate for exchange. It is marked by willingness to consider, in the name of prevention, ideas and strategies that at first may offend us. We have to work constantly, in other words, at changing those attitudes that feed the infection, at keeping open minds as well as open hearts.

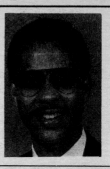

Dr. Reed Tuckson
YOU CAN MAKE MY JOB EASIER

Dr. Reed Tuckson is the commissioner of public health for the District of Columbia.

I AM CONVINCED that when the history of this time is written, it will be best characterized by how we as a society responded to the multiple challenges presented to us by AIDS. Few issues present such a variety of individual and collective choices to problems that, while basic to the human experience, are complex in their implications and offer few easy solutions. This, combined with the growing realization that the lives of many thousands of our citizens are at stake, demands that we all work together to conduct an effective, competent, and principled struggle to preserve the lives of our citizens. In so doing, we preserve that which is best about us as people.

As the Commissioner of Public Health for a major city, I have a responsibility to provide leadership in developing and implementing the public policy response to this epidemic. As a citizen, I share with every other American the responsibility to protect our own individual health and to participate in an informed and compassionate manner in the shaping of our collective local, state, and national behavior.

Ultimately, our success will depend heavily on cooperation between the American people and the professional public health community. I am happy to have this opportunity to suggest ways that you can make it easier for people in jobs like mine to better serve you and this country in this emergency:

• You should learn the facts about how AIDS is transmitted and how it is *not* transmitted. It is tragic to lose lives because of ignorance and misinformation. It is equally tragic for us to make incorrect choices that harm others because of this same ignorance and misinformation.

• Share that knowledge with your family and community. Invite public-health professionals to address your church and community organizations. Parents have a special responsibility to talk with their children and advise them about the consequences of their behavior in a manner that is sensitive to both the child's age and the family's values.

• Many cities need community-based treatment centers for drug users and homes for persons with AIDS who cannot care for themselves but don't need to be hospitalized. It is difficult enough to provide such services without facing neighborhood opposition. This is a critical moment in the history of this country; it is time to draw together, not push each other away.

• Beware of any discriminatory actions directed against persons with AIDS or persons who are infected with the virus. If people are concerned that their HIV status (that is, whether they carry the human immunodeficiency virus) could result in the loss of their home or job, could cause their child to be denied access to an education, or could subject them to the scorn of their neighbors, then people at risk will be reluctant to cooperate with the public-health system.

• Many communities need volunteers to assist in AIDS-related work. Offering to help with simple chores such as shopping or housecleaning could be of enormous benefit to the person with AIDS and to the community in general.

• Finally, too many babies born to infected mothers are condemned to confinement in our nation's hospitals. We need foster parents and other people of goodwill to volunteer to care for these precious little lives.

When the history of our time is written, let America be proud that we responded to our challenges in a competent and compassionate manner. Let it record the collective effort of a society that expressed the noblest qualities of its civilization.

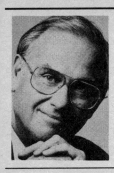

Senator Lowell Weicker, Jr.
WRITE YOUR ELECTED OFFICIALS

Senator Lowell Weicker, Jr., (R-Conn.) served in the U.S. Senate from 1971 to 1988. There, as ranking member of the Senate Appropriations Subcommittee on Labor, Health and Human Services, and Education, he was an outspoken advocate for AIDS research and education programs.

A FEELING OF POWERLESSNESS in the face of the AIDS crisis is common. After all, if the experts can't decide how to address it, what can the average person do? But there is one kind of power all Americans have by virtue of our form of government: political power. Use it; contact your representatives.

You don't need to be a highly paid, professional lobbyist to make a mark on AIDS spending or policy. Every constituent call is listened to. Every letter is read. Even if these contacts do not change the officeholder's mind or vote, they send the crucial message that somebody cares.

Uncertainty as to how best to address a member of Congress or advance an argument should not keep you from putting pen to paper. Etiquette and sophistication are not the issue. The need for a concerted federal response to AIDS is. And that won't come without a fight.

Every month, as many as ten thousand people wrote my Washington office on virtually every subject imaginable, from how to obtain Social Security checks to what to do about the wild horses and burros running loose on public lands out west.

Some letters arrive on elegant, letterhead stationery, meticulously typed. Others are hastily handwritten on a legal pad. As long as they are legible, they are read.

Those about AIDS have focused on almost every aspect of the crisis, including: the development of cures, vaccines, and life-prolonging drugs; the debate over whether to base our educational efforts on the scientific consensus of our public-health experts or the philosophical agenda of some in government; legislation to protect the civil rights of those who test positive for the AIDS virus; the search for ways to care for AIDS patients in a manner more compassionate and less costly; and just how terrible it is to watch someone you love die from AIDS.

Certain qualities make some kinds of mail more effective than others. Hundreds of mass-produced postcards may well lack the impact of one personalized statement of concern. AIDS has yet to be made real to many in government, despite all the headlines. A constituent's first-hand experience with the disease can help bridge the gap between AIDS in the abstract and AIDS as an everyday matter of life and death.

Keeping abreast of what is happening on AIDS issues in Congress can make for a better timed and targeted appeal. Budgets for research, education, and treatment are hammered out over a matter of months. Other battles — such as one last year over an amendment to restrict the flow of federally funded AIDS information to the gay community — often materialize overnight. Most news media cover AIDS closely. Citizens' action groups make it their business to monitor developments even more intensively and to get that information out to the interested public.

Along with the constitutional right to tell your legislators what you think comes a responsibility to study and think about the issues you're writing about. A wide range of responses to the AIDS epidemic have been proposed by various individuals and organizations. Some of these responses make sense. Others, while they may sound appealing at first, would simply make the problem worse, or would create other problems without stopping the spread of AIDS. In the next chapter, the former Surgeon General of the United States looks at some of the measures that are — and are not — called for.

In addition to your own members of Congress, consider contacting others who serve on committees and subcommittees that authorize AIDS legislation or appropriate AIDS funds. Admittedly, mail from out-of-state voters may not carry the weight of a constituent's letter, but at the very least it is a reminder that AIDS is a problem that respects no borders. It is a national threat demanding a national response.

Dr. C. Everett Koop
LOOKING TO THE FUTURE

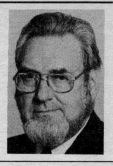

Dr. C. Everett Koop was the Surgeon General of the United States from 1981 to 1989. During that time he earned widespread praise for his handling of the AIDS crisis.

MY REPORT ON acquired immune deficiency syndrome, released in October of 1986, contains the information on AIDS that most Americans need to know about this disease. If I were to release it today, it would contain the same information. I encourage you to get a copy of this report and read it.

There has often been controversy about what action is needed to stop the spread of AIDS. Some proposals, such as compulsory blood testing, quarantine, and identification of AIDS carriers by some visible sign, largely reflect a lack of knowledge about AIDS. Our efforts must go into other areas, the most important of which are discussed below.

Education: Education concerning AIDS must start at the lowest grade possible as part of any health and hygiene program. This education should be in the context of respect for our bodies and the need for caring, kind, considerate, and lasting relationships. The appearance of AIDS could bring together diverse groups of parents and educators with opposing views on inclusion of sex education in the curricula.

General sex education in schools should begin in the third grade, with AIDS-specific materials introduced in middle school or junior high school. There is now no doubt that we need sex education in schools and that it must include information on heterosexual and homosexual relationships. The threat of AIDS should be sufficient to permit a sex-education curriculum with a heavy emphasis on prevention of AIDS and other sexually transmitted diseases.

Compulsory Blood Testing: Compulsory blood testing of individuals is not necessary. The procedure could be unmanageable and cost prohibitive. It can be expected that many who *test* negatively might actually be positive due to *recent* exposure to the AIDS virus and give a false sense of security to the individual and his or her sexual partners concerning necessary protective behavior. Proper prevention behavior will protect the American public and contain the AIDS epidemic. A single screening of a low-prevalence group will show many people as positive who, on further testing, will prove to be negative. What is really needed is the anonymous testing of a sample of low-risk people to get an estimate of the problem.

Quarantine: Quarantine has no role in the management of AIDS because AIDS is not spread by casual contact. The only time that some form of quarantine might be indicated is in a situation where an individual carrying the AIDS virus knowingly and willingly continues to expose others through sexual contact or sharing drug equipment. Such circumstances should be managed on a case-by-case basis by local authorities.

Identification of AIDS Carriers by Some Visible Sign: Those who suggest the marking of carriers of the AIDS virus by some visible sign, such as a tattoo, have not thought the matter through thoroughly. It would require testing of the entire population, which is unnecessary, unmanageable, and costly. It would miss those recently infected individuals who would test negatively, but be infected. The entire procedure would give a false sense of security. AIDS must be treated as a disease that can infect anyone. AIDS should not be used as an excuse to discriminate against any group or individual.

Confidentiality: Because of the stigma that has been associated with AIDS, many afflicted with the disease or who are infected with the AIDS virus are reluctant to be identified with AIDS. Because there is no vaccine to prevent AIDS and no cure, many feel there is nothing to be gained by revealing sexual contacts that might also be infected with the AIDS virus. When a community or a state requires reporting of those infected with the AIDS virus to public-health authorities in order to trace sexual and intravenous-drug contacts — as is the practice with other sexually transmitted diseases — those infected with the AIDS virus go underground out of the mainstream of health care and education. For this reason current public-health practice is to protect the privacy of the individual infected with the AIDS virus and to maintain the strictest confidentiality concerning his or her health records.

Discrimination against People with AIDS: Many individuals who have AIDS are nonetheless able to live reasonably normal lives. The same is true of those who carry HIV (the human immunodeficiency virus) but have not shown symptoms of the disease.

Because AIDS is not spread through casual contact, there is no reason why these people should face discrimination of any sort as they attempt to live their day-to-day lives. Enlightened policies by businesses and employers, combined with existing anti-discrimination laws, should ensure that such discrimination does not become a problem. If that is not sufficient, however, further legislation may be necessary.

FOLLOW-UP:

The Surgeon General's Report on AIDS is published in both English and Spanish editions. You can get a free copy by calling the National AIDS Information Clearinghouse: 1-800-342-2437.

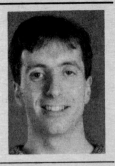

Kevin George

SUPPORT YOUR LOCAL AIDS GROUP

Kevin George is a native Bostonian who devotes much of his time to martial arts, which he has studied for nine years, and politics. He is active in PWA organizations in Boston.

WHEN I WAS DIAGNOSED with AIDS in March 1987, I was a restaurant manager. After my diagnosis, I was forced to go on Social Security so I could get the health benefits I needed.

Since then I have moved three times, and now I live in Boston to be near my family. Living in rural areas as well as major cities has made me acutely aware of the need for services for people with AIDS in every part of the country.

To provide any type of service costs money. For the person with AIDS (PWA), there is often no place to go to for help but the local AIDS service organization. Not only do donations keep the doors open, but the money given helps people with AIDS in many different ways.

One pressing need is direct financial assistance to people with AIDS or pre-AIDS conditions. Government social agencies have strict guidelines for defining AIDS. Often a person will have ARC (AIDS-Related Complex) and be unable to work, but will not have all the symptoms required to get financial assistance. This is where AIDS groups often can do the greatest good. Donations provide immediate help for the person with ARC — money to pay rent and other bills, and to buy food and medicine until he or she can get government benefits.

Donations to your local AIDS organization also can supply medical aid to people with AIDS and ARC when programs like Medicaid won't cover treatment.

Local AIDS groups, usually through a combination of volunteers and paid staff, offer a wide range of services to PWAs. These services often include transportation to appointments, housecleaning, shopping, meal preparation, laundry, social excursions, and personal services such as haircuts and massages and peer counseling. Although they may seem minor, services like these are what keeps a person with AIDS going.

A haircut gives a tremendous ego boost. A massage gives a wonderful sense of relief to a person desperate for human contact. A ride to the doctor is important but more important is the fact that a friendly face is waiting in the reception area to share the good news of a medical improvement or the bad news of a downturn. These services couldn't exist without both volunteer help and financial contributions to pay the overhead.

AIDS organizations often provide psychological counseling as well. Getting that first AIDS diagnosis is a frightening experience. In the beginning, just someone to talk to can be the most important need a person with AIDS has.

Many AIDS organizations also offer counseling and support groups. Some provide social services like weekly dinners for PWAs.

Strong support services can make a crucial difference in the health and sanity of a PWA. Unfortunately, a local shortage of such services has forced many PWAs to relocate. That means they have to give up friends, loved ones, and a known environment. It would be so much better if every city could gather the resources to provide these services.

For me, the help and services I received from local AIDS groups were invaluable. But probably the greatest impact of these was the knowledge that every time I received aid, I knew I was receiving the support of another human being. I realized that I was not alone in fighting this disease. My sense of isolation was lessened every time a stranger reached out a hand. Even the smallest gift of time helped push back the fear and the negative feelings.

People with AIDS are human beings who need to know that someone still cares. Whether you give money, or time, or both, it does make a difference.

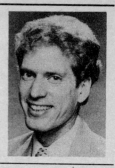

Jeffrey Zaslow
EDUCATION DOESN'T HAPPEN ONLY IN SCHOOLS

Jeffrey Zaslow began his writing career with the Orlando Sentinel *and the* Wall Street Journal. *In 1987, after a highly publicized nationwide search, the Chicago* Sun-Times *selected him to replace Ann Landers; his column "All That Zazz" is now syndicated to over forty newspapers.*

YOU'RE AT A PARTY and a friend tells a "gay" joke with an AIDS punchline. You're at your folks' home for Thanksgiving and some relatives argue that any homosexual who gets AIDS "deserves it." Or maybe your neighbors are pressuring you to sign a petition seeking the dismissal of a schoolteacher suspected of having AIDS.

In the course of such day-to-day social interactions, you may meet people who are paranoid, misinformed, ignorant, or just plain scared about AIDS. As an advice columnist, I hear from and about such people all the time. And there are things all of us can do to help clear up misconceptions, and to respond sensitively to insensitive remarks.

The best way to help the naive and the uninformed is to encourage them to educate themselves. Resist the urge to angrily set them straight in front of others. Often, it's best to take them aside and have a friendly chat about your concerns. When someone tells a tasteless joke or makes an anti-gay comment that suggests AIDS-phobia, you might respond: "AIDS is still a mystery in some ways, but there are a lot of things about the disease that are known. From what I've read, I've learned that ... "

You may be dealing with a seriously uninformed person. For instance, I got a letter from a reader whose 65-year-old friend is sexually active with several partners. "She believes that, at her age, she cannot contract AIDS," the reader wrote. "No one has been able to convince her that old age doesn't make you immune to the disease. Those of us who love her are concerned. How can we caution her?"

The advice I gave: "Go to the library, photocopy articles about AIDS, and give them to her. A librarian can steer you to many books and articles that clearly answer typical questions and refute common myths about the disease."

Misinformation about AIDS results in different responses from different people. A mother wrote to tell me about her son and daughter, both in their twenties, who say that AIDS is a disease almost everyone will have in the future. "They say there are all sorts of ways to get AIDS, even through insect bites, and that the government has covered up these facts so there isn't a panic," the mother wrote. "As a result, my children believe it doesn't matter whether they are sexually careful or not. They are behaving in bold ways — as if there's no tomorrow."

If someone you know is equally fatalistic — or has an irrational fear of infection — don't be afraid to bring up the topic of safe sex. Just tell them the facts, as you know them, without being preachy or accusatory, and offer to bring them written material about AIDS. They can then read up on the disease at their leisure.

I've gotten letters from people asking if they can get AIDS from masturbation, shaking hands, hot tubs, or riding on elevators with people carrying the AIDS virus. (Indeed, a Los Angeles *Times* poll indicates that ten percent of Americans believe AIDS can be contracted by handling money.) I encourage all of them to call the National AIDS Hotline (1-800-

342-2437), where counselors gladly answer questions and mail out free information.

Some people have misguided notions about how to respond to the growing number of people with AIDS. Refute their suggestions only after acknowledging their fears. For instance, one letter writer to my column suggested that a school be opened for children with the AIDS virus: "People with AIDS who are still able to work could teach these kids. The kids and the teachers could come from all over the country. That way, normal people in schools wouldn't be infected."

I responded that herding kids into a leper-colony-style school would be cruel and unnecessary. I quoted the federal Centers for Disease Control, which recommends that students with AIDS continue going to their schools because the risk to others appears "nonexistent." I also acknowledged the fears that led to the proposal: "Yes, we must make sure that children with AIDS don't infect other kids. Safeguards and school policies must be studied. But any solution must be a humane one."

The best way to help inform others about AIDS is to stay informed yourself. When you come across groundbreaking or explanatory articles about AIDS, save them for future reference. If you're knowledgeable about AIDS, you'll sound authoritative. And never be afraid to discuss the disease. Talking leads to understanding.

2

EVERYONE
CAN MAKE
A DIFFERENCE

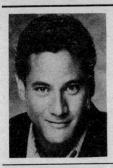

Greg Louganis
BE A
BUDDY

Greg Louganis is a two-time Olympic gold medal diving champion and has won 43 U.S. National titles in diving.

BEING A FRIEND to a person with AIDS has been a rewarding, positive experience for me. It's the best way I know how to make a difference in the fight against AIDS. And it's something every one of us can do, regularly and enjoyably, without too much difficulty.

Although I haven't participated in an actual "buddy program," the things I've done to help my friend Ryan White are based on similar principles of reaching out to those who are struggling with the disease, offering love, support, and companionship when they need it most. Not only does it make me feel better for trying to help, it helps the person who has AIDS immeasurably.

I first heard about Ryan White while watching a news report on CNN. A sixteen-year-old boy with severe hemophilia, Ryan got AIDS from a batch of blood-clotting factor that was contaminated with the virus. Because he had AIDS, he'd been barred from attending school in his hometown of Kokomo, Indiana. Many local parents were afraid their kids would get AIDS, too. But Ryan White chose to stand up for himself — to fight for his right to attend school. I was impressed by the guy's drive and determination.

In many ways I identified with his struggle. When I went

to school, people constantly made fun of me because I was dark, and I was dyslexic. I was always being called derogatory names. If I'd been asked not to come back to school, that would have been fine with me. But Ryan White wanted to go to school so badly he was willing to go to court and fight to be allowed back in. I looked upon his pursuit of an education the way I look at my pursuit of diving. He was fully committed to a goal. I admire that.

So when I realized the national diving championships were being held in Indiana, I contacted Ryan and invited him to come and watch the various competitions. I wanted to share something of myself with him, and to let him know how much he had inspired me. It was a great experience for both of us — and the start of a warm, special friendship.

I try to see Ryan and his family as often as I can. Last year he was able to come out to Malibu and stay with me for a while. He said he was ready to move in, except for the earthquakes. He's not too crazy about earthquakes, and while he was here we had a pretty big one.

Living so far apart from Ryan, it's hard to be with him as much as I would like. I use the telephone to make contact. When he turned sixteen last December, I called and was delighted to discover that a lot of his school friends had dropped by and were having a party for him. Since he moved to Cicero, Indiana, things have been much better for Ryan and his family. The people in Cicero are really supportive, and because of all the media coverage, Ryan's become something of a celebrity in town. Best of all, Ryan has an incredible family who take great care of him.

Ryan White is the first person with AIDS I've ever dealt with directly. And it's been a terrific opportunity for me to help him in any way I can. I realize, even more than before, how little there is to fear in working with and assisting people who have this disease. It only takes a moment to lift someone's spirits. Whenever we're together, Ryan and I discuss his treatment, and how he's reacting to the various medications he's taking. He's on AZT now, and seems to be responding very well. But I know it must be pretty hard on him. We talk about his energy level. That's real important. Most of the time, he tells me how school is going. That's number one with him. His report card is always full of A's.

The thing I respect most about Ryan is that someone in his position could be very angry or bitter. But he isn't. He's very accepting. He's taken the positive road, eager to educate people about AIDS and about his predicament. In spite of his own difficulties, he's trying to help others. I don't know if I could react with the same degree of strength and character if I were in his position. The truth is I've learned so much from this little kid — this brave young man. I'm proud to be his friend.

If you want to help someone with AIDS, one way to start is by looking into your neighborhood AIDS hotline or task force. I recommend that you learn more about what it takes to be a buddy before casually helping a stranger, or even a close friend who is sick with AIDS, because dealing with a fatal disease is never simple. As other "buddies" have told me, it helps to work with a team or a support group who can share the psychological and emotional load. Yet, there is no reason to delay making contact and letting someone know you care. Even a simple card can brighten someone's day.

By working together, we can all help others who have AIDS find comfort and dignity even in the most difficult of circumstances.

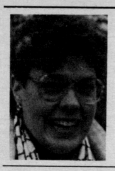

Kate Capps
VOLUNTEER YOUR TIME

Kate Capps is the marketing manager at Ohio State University Press, and a volunteer with the Columbus AIDS Task Force.

IN THE SUMMER OF 1985, a casual acquaintance of mine died of AIDS. His death affected me more than I expected it to. I was angry, upset, and suddenly, worried for some of my friends. I felt compelled to do something even though I felt no personal risk. How could I help stop a possible epidemic?

My opportunity arose in the fall when I heard about the Columbus (Ohio) AIDS Task Force. My volunteer work began with an intensive weekend of training which prepared me to be a "buddy" or helpmate to a person with AIDS (PWA). The training also helped me to decide whether I could handle being a buddy or whether I should find another way to help. I learned about the disease itself and about what to expect when working one-on-one with a PWA or PWArc (person with AIDS-related complex).

Being a buddy requires a special commitment, and it is just one of the ways that you can help. Our task force is involved in a variety of activities, and almost all are carried out by volunteers. These activities can be divided into direct-contact and non-contact tasks, enabling us to feel comfortable about our participation. Most of the activities require only time and understanding.

One of the simplest, safest, and most important things I

do is give blood through the American Red Cross. I cannot contract AIDS by giving blood, and people in high-risk categories can no longer donate blood, which means reduced numbers of donors. In addition, PWAs often need transfusions.

In Columbus, some task force volunteers staff an AIDS telephone hotline providing accurate information to anyone who calls. Some write grant proposals for funding. Others provide their secretarial and word-processing skills for correspondence and mailing-list updates; writing and producing a monthly newsletter and flyers; and stuffing and mailing those materials. If someone needs to work at home, materials for these projects can be delivered and picked up by another volunteer. Some people participate in the task force speakers bureau, helping to educate various groups.

Our task force has monthly meetings known as in-service sessions for volunteers, to keep them abreast of current information on AIDS and to provide them with useful information and support in their roles as buddies. People involved in helping professions, such as nursing, law, medicine, or psychology, address volunteers on a variety of subjects from home nursing care to bereavement to the influence of drugs and alcohol on PWAs' health.

Other volunteers help to staff the HIV test center. At this anonymous blood-testing facility, volunteers are trained to take information from people desiring to be tested and to counsel people concerning the ramifications of the test results. Working at the test center requires some personal inner strength and sensitivity, because you will be telling people whether or not they have contracted a deadly virus. You'll need to be prepared to react sensitively to a wide range of possible responses.

Being a buddy can be one of the more difficult of the volunteer activities. It is an open-ended commitment to an individual who will be depending on you, and it means direct contact with someone who is terminally ill. Your involvement can be as simple as weekly phone calls or visits, or providing a ride to the store or a doctor's appointment. It can also mean more involvement depending on the PWA's needs — grocery shopping, errand running, light housework, or, in extreme cases, home nursing care. If a PWA needs constant care, a buddy group may be formed. I would not recommend being a buddy without some educational training to find out how you feel about working closely with someone who has AIDS. Your own feelings and fears about death may surface in ways that surprise you.

I have been a buddy twice during the last three years, and for me it required a commitment to provide time and care. It was a strangely rewarding experience, because I learned about living, dying, and unconditional love from someone terminally ill, and in return I helped each to live the last year of his life as much on his own terms as possible.

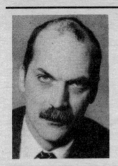

John Preston
LITTLE EXTRAS THAT MAKE A DIFFERENCE

John Preston is a sex-education counselor, lecturer, and author (Hot Living *and* Safe Sex). *He is the writer-in-residence of The AIDS Project, Portland, Maine.*

KRIS, A FRIEND OF MINE who's a PWA (person with AIDS), sometimes had trouble finding solid foods he could eat. For a short period of time, it seemed the only thing he could enjoy was Häagen-Dazs ice cream. It was something that certainly wasn't in his budget. Since it was important during those couple of days that he get anything he could into his stomach, I gladly brought him as many regular deliveries of Häagen-Dazs as he would eat. If what he could use was premium-quality — and premium-priced — dessert, then so be it; he had the right to have it.

Later, after that crisis was passed, I realized that Häagen-Dazs had another purpose in his life. That small luxury made a great difference in Kris's attitude; it provided a symbol to him of the pleasure of food beyond subsistence; its heavy creaminess was a simple totem of how good life could be. I realized then that providing money for Häagen-Dazs for Kris was a worthwhile priority.

There are lots of ways to spend money, and there are many conflicting needs, but that impressed on me the special added value that some items can bring to a person's quality of life.

Research and organizational work are vital, and the

groups that support them need your donations, there's no question about it. But we can't forget that the AIDS crisis involves people and that any bureaucracy, no matter how benign, has to make group decisions that sometimes leave out individuality or the extra touch.

Faced with an often long and debilitating battle that usually uses up any discretionary income that might once have been available, the PWA doesn't always have access to the small extras that can often make such a difference in one's attitude and well-being.

If your local organizations collect food for PWAs, make sure there are some special gourmet items in the basket you give. Granted, some people will have special dietary needs, but even the most restricted diets can often accommodate special taste treats, if you find out just what the limitations are for an individual. Some library research can show you what options you might help bring into the person's life. (And the cookbook you discover might well be a special donation you might want to make to the next food drive.)

When you answer a request for clothing from an organization, stop and think that an especially well-made, bright piece of clothing with a flair to its design and appearance might add something to a collection of utilitarian pieces.

A drama buff might really appreciate a ticket to a theater performance. A reader might long for the luxury of a hardcover edition of a new book by a favorite author. A dinner at one of the really good restaurants in town might be the best medicine another person could ever receive.

If you don't know PWAs, deliver that kind of special gift to your local AIDS organization along with your donation for general support. Ask someone who works with PWAs if there's something special you could offer in addition to the help you're providing organizations. Most such workers won't have to think long before coming up with someone who would really benefit from a unique offering. The gleam in that staffer's eyes will tell you that he or she knows the right person.

Representative Henry Waxman

THE URGENT NEED FOR RESEARCH

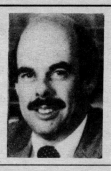

Congressman Henry Waxman (D-Calif.) is chairman of the House Health and Environment subcommittee. He is a leading proponent of increased spending for AIDS research, and the prime sponsor of a bill calling for voluntary testing, confidentiality, and non-discrimination.

RESEARCHERS SAY THAT they learned a valuable lesson from their early efforts during the polio epidemic: Look for a vaccine first and for a better iron lung later. Fighting a war from the wrong front sacrifices time and lives.

For the AIDS epidemic, we must adopt a new strategy. We have to look for a cause, a vaccine, a treatment, and a cure — all at the same time. Fighting only a one-front war would sacrifice time and lives. There are so many people already infected that we cannot simply wait for a vaccine.

It's a hard lesson. To carry on a multi-front effort against a new disease requires more people and more money than we are accustomed to spending.

But without such an effort, we will stand by as the number of Americans with AIDS grows and as their health-care costs skyrocket. These health costs will be borne by every taxpayer and every purchaser of health insurance. If research can limit the number of people who develop AIDS or even the number of illnesses they get, the research will pay for itself dozens of times over.

In a time of tight budgets, however, this simple equation — research can save lives and money — often gets lost in the debate about federal spending. The pressures to slow even the most fundamental research and public-health programs are enormous, and the competing calls to cut taxes or spend scarce money on other programs are loud.

To be sure that AIDS research and public-health programs remain strong, concerned people must make their voices heard above these calls and support federal AIDS research efforts.

Private organizations have also been crucial in AIDS research. The American Foundation for AIDS Research (AmFAR) has supported many research projects, often with immediate funds for projects that the government has not undertaken. AmFAR has also created a public awareness of the need for greater federal activity. Other groups, such as the American Cancer Society and the American Lung Association, are beginning to recognize that AIDS programs require their help as well and that AIDS research will produce spinoffs in dealing with other diseases. Some local AIDS groups — such as the Community Research Initiative in New York — also work with physicians and researchers on scientific projects and information exchange.

Letters to Congress will be noticed and answered. Your contributions to private organizations can multiply that effect. If we are to win this war, we must support it.

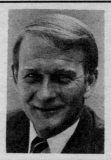

Jody Powell
WORKING WITH THE MEDIA

Jody Powell was the White House Press Secretary under President Jimmy Carter. Since then he has been a news analyst for ABC News and a syndicated columnist; he is now the chairman of Ogilvy & Mather Public Affairs.

THE BEST WAY TO STOP the spread of AIDS is with information. That's why people need to know the facts about how the disease is transmitted. They also need to understand that casual contact with a person with AIDS is perfectly safe. And since most of the information the American public receives about AIDS comes from newspapers or television, the media has a very important job to do — with your help.

As we've seen far too many times already, people who don't know the facts about AIDS are also more likely to have irrational fears. These fears lead to situations where young children are unnecessarily prevented from attending school, and critically ill people are discriminated against cruelly.

That's why it's so important that the media do all it can to educate the public in a calm and responsible way. News coverage about the disease has to be complete, factual, and unbiased. If it's not, some people may not change behavior that can put them at risk. Others will continue to shun people with the disease who need support and acceptance more ever before.

One of the most important things you can do about AIDS

in your community, then, is to work with the media to make sure their coverage is accurate and thorough. Reporters aren't perfect: they are usually facing tight deadlines, and don't always have the time and medical expertise to prepare themselves adequately to cover the issue. Sometimes a reporter may have to cover an AIDS-related story without much prior experience in the subject.

One of the best ways to measure how effectively local media is covering the AIDS issue is to be on the lookout for certain "buzz words" that are still used by many reporters. These include:

Bodily fluids: One of the most confusing phrases used in discussions of AIDS transmission, it should never be used without a detailed explanation of which bodily fluids actually contain the HIV virus in concentrations sufficient to transmit the disease. Small wonder so many parents were afraid that their children could be exposed to the virus through casual contact. Sweat, saliva, and tears are all bodily fluids, but do not carry a threat of HIV infection. Reports on AIDS should make it clear that semen, vaginal fluids, and blood are the concern here.

General population: This misnomer artificially divides the American people into those who have the disease and those who do not. Everyone who has AIDS — regardless of sexual orientation, race, gender, or how they were exposed to the virus — is part of the "general population."

High-risk groups: This misleading and potentially discriminatory term implies that some kind of demographic trait, rather than behavioral practice, is responsible for AIDS exposure. "High-risk behavior," on the other hand, is a perfectly appropriate term.

AIDS victims: People with AIDS are not victims; they are people struggling to live normal lives in the face of a fatal disease. We don't refer to people with other diseases as victims, and shouldn't make that mistake with people with AIDS. The most preferable phrase is "people with AIDS."

AIDS virus vs. AIDS: Many people still confuse exposure to the HIV virus with the disease itself. More than one million people in the United States are believed to have been exposed to the virus; about one hundred thousand actual cases have been reported. Coverage should always explain the difference.

Condoms: Reports recommending condom use to reduce the risk of HIV exposure should clearly state that latex condoms with a spermicide are preferable (natural lamb condoms may not provide the necessary protection).

Intimate sexual contact: This is a polite phrase that doesn't tell the reader anything useful (many people regard kissing and fondling as intimate). Certain sexual practices — especially unprotected anal intercourse — are known to pose a much greater chance of HIV transmission than others. News articles should make this clear.

If you find that local coverage of AIDS is not all that it should be, do something about it. In many instances you may actually find that you know more than the reporter covering the story. Nine times out of ten the reporter responsible will appreciate your interest and assistance.

Become familiar with all area reporters who regularly cover AIDS stories, as well as their editors and producers. If there is a problem with a specific story, contact the reporter involved and explain your concerns in a positive way. Don't be confrontational; simply point out the problem and offer to provide information that will help improve future coverage.

Always be specific when voicing your concerns — be ready to point out factual errors, or examples of alarmist, biased, or incomplete reporting. Encourage other observers who share your concern about local coverage to express their views as well. Write letters to the editor, or write an opinion article for the editorial pages.

I learned the power of the media first hand when I was at the White House. The media is and will remain a critical link in our efforts to educate the American public on the facts about AIDS, and how to halt its transmission. Responsible reporting provides one of our best hopes of making the public understand that AIDS is everyone's concern, and an issue that affects every community.

Cleve Jones
THE NAMES PROJECT

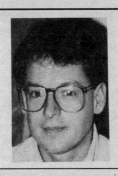

Cleve Jones has been active in gay community politics for over a decade. He began The Names Project in 1987 to memorialize people who have died of AIDS.

I WAS DEVASTATED when my best friend was killed by AIDS in the autumn of 1986. Marvin and I had been friends, roommates, and travel companions at various times over the previous fourteen years. Our friendship survived long separations and the many upheavals of our lives; we planned the future of our lives together. Although we were separated by a continent for most of his eighteen-month struggle against AIDS, we communicated regularly, and I was able to be with him during the last weeks of his life at his parents' home in Rhode Island. Marvin died on October 10, 1986.

In the months that followed, I found myself resisting an increasing sense of despair. Marvin's memory was so hard-edged and painful that I found it difficult to maintain my day-to-day life. On a clear day in February, my friend Joseph Durant and I spread lengths of fabric across my back patio and began painting names with some leftover spray paint we found in the garage; I painted the thirteen letters of Marvin Feldman with black paint and stencil. The background was a jumble of grey and blue triangular shadows with pink and blue triangles overlaid to form six-pointed stars.

Joseph painted a smoky, rust-colored sky. He then

plunged his bare feet in gold paint and danced across the fabric, leaving golden footprints over the name of choreographer Ed Mock.

Neither of us was particularly satisfied with the results, but for several hours we talked, laughed, and exchanged anecdotes about our lost friends. I found myself able to focus clearly on Marvin's life, his character and personality. By the end of the afternoon I felt a deeper understanding of our friendship and an even greater gratitude for having been able to share so much of my life with him.

When I realized how important this process had been for me, I started suggesting to other people that they join me in making a giant quilt. A few months later, people from all over started sending me fabric panels that they had made for their friends, lovers, sons, and daughters. I was embarrassed that they were all so much more beautiful than the panel I made for Marvin; but soon other friends made wonderful panels for him, and I stopped worrying about mine. Now I think even mine is all right.

I still miss Marvin and all my other friends who have been taken by this hideous disease. The quilt helps me to hold their memories close to my heart in a form that comforts me and strengthens my resolve.

The quilt now consists of almost eleven thousand panels. Millions have viewed it on television, and hundreds of thousands have entered its fabric walkways, but the heart and soul of the quilt resides in homes across the country when friends and families gather to sew together their memories of love.

HOW TO CREATE A MEMORIAL PANEL:

1. Select a durable, lightweight fabric for the background. Cut and hem the fabric to 3' by 6'. (We'll hem it for you if you leave 3 inches extra fabric on each side.)

2. Design the panel. Use lettering, pictures, and other artwork in whatever way you like. Some suggestions:
Appliqué: sew letters to background fabric.
Painting: brush design on with paint, dye, or ink.
Stencil: spray paint cut-out letters or design.
Collage: glue on material with fabric glue.
Embroider: sew on beads, sequins, or rhinestones.

3. When the panel is complete, write a one- or two-page description of the person you have memorialized. Enclose a photograph of the person if you're willing to part with it.

4. Wrap the panel securely before mailing it to: The Names Project, P. O. Box 14573, San Francisco, CA 94114.

5. Please include as generous a contribution as you can.

Have any questions? Call The Names Project at 415-863-5511.

John-Manuel Andriote
SHOW YOUR APPRECIATION

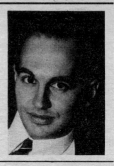

John-Manuel Andriote has written for a variety of publications ranging from The Christian Science Monitor *to* The Advocate, *and has served as publicist for the National AIDS Network.*

I WAS FORTUNATE during my college days to have as a mentor a professor I respected and admired. After I graduated, we began a correspondence. In one of his letters, my professor friend told me that whatever I chose to do with my life, I must never neglect what he said was an ability to write beautifully. His words stuck with me. His encouragement propelled me to explore a career as a writer. In the years since I got that letter I've acquired a master's degree in journalism and pursued a career as an author of newspaper and magazine articles. Those words of support meant a lot.

Writing about AIDS, being a friend to a number of people who are living with or have succumbed to AIDS, I have become aware of a worldwide network of individuals who are involved first-hand with the AIDS epidemic. Some are on the front lines, providing services to people with AIDS; others are providing support behind the scenes. AIDS has brought forward people who understand the healing power of unity, and the insidious nature of fear and divisiveness.

People like former Surgeon General C. Everett Koop, who took bold personal and political risks to counter fear and promote a rational response to AIDS.

Researchers who labor away in the laboratories of the country's universities and research centers, searching for a vaccine, hoping for a cure.

Politicians who endorse legislation that treats AIDS as a public-health problem requiring compassion and medically sound policy, rather than a moral problem to be inveighed against from on high.

Religious leaders who place compassion above dogma.

Physicians who strive to heal, but who find themselves too often feeling impotent in the presence of a disease that has killed so many previously healthy young people.

Reporters who dog public officials — and often their editors — to be sure AIDS is kept on the agenda of priority issues.

The many thousands of volunteers in community clinics, hospitals, and social-service agencies who donate countless hours operating local AIDS hotlines, preparing meals, or doing the grocery shopping for people too ill to do it themselves, lending an ear, offering a hug or a smile.

All these people stand out to me as models of what is best in the human spirit. Most of these people do their work out of personal conviction. Like Dr. Rieux in Albert Camus's novel *The Plague*, they contribute their time and skills because it's the right, humane thing to do. It simply *has* to be done. They're not after applause and awards. They are after fair and dignified treatment for others who often can't defend their own right to it. It's hard work.

In October 1987, the National AIDS Network (NAN) honored some ninety AIDS volunteers from across the nation with a ceremony dedicated to them and to all "Americans Who Care." Those who were honored remarked how appreciated they felt, and how inspired. Inspired to go home and resume their work and commitment.

NAN's ceremony was a formal way of doing something we all can do easily enough — showing appreciation to people who are battling AIDS and caring for those it has afflicted.

Sending a note to your local AIDS clinic is one way. Encouraging your elected officials to endorse a compassionate response to AIDS, then thanking them when they do, is another. A word of encouragement or note to an AIDS researcher you've read of in the newspaper, or a co-worker who does AIDS-related volunteer work, can really brighten that person's day. It can give them the energy to keep going, even if the going gets tough.

The seventeenth-century poet John Donne wrote that "No man is an island." The AIDS epidemic proves once again the truth of Donne's words — our need to stand together, to encourage one another, in a common battle and a shared humanity. I know personally how far a word of encouragement goes. I'm certain your encouragement would mean a great deal to people who have dedicated themselves to eradicating AIDS and ensuring the dignity of the people it has affected.

**Dixie Beckham,
Luis Palacios,
Vincent Patti, and
Michael Shernoff**

WHEN A FRIEND HAS AIDS

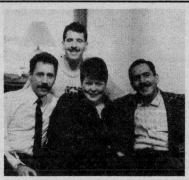

---

*The authors have worked together at Chelsea Psychotherapy
Associates, a group practice in Manhattan. They are also volunteers at Gay Men's Health Crisis, the world's oldest AIDS
service-provider organization.*

WHEN SOMEONE YOU KNOW becomes ill, especially with a
serious illness like AIDS, it's easy to feel helpless or inadequate. Here are some thoughts and suggestions that can help
you to help someone who is very ill.

• Try not to avoid your friend. Be there — it instills hope.
Be the friend, the loved one you've always been, especially now
when it is most important.

• Touch your friend. A simple squeeze of the hand or a
hug can let him know that you still care. You cannot contract
AIDS by simply touching — and hugs are very reassuring.

• Call and ask if it is okay to come for a visit. Let your
friend make the decision. If she doesn't feel up to a visitor that
day, you can visit on another occasion. Now is a time when your
friendship can help keep loneliness and fear at a distance.

• Call and say you'd like to bring a favorite dish. Ask what
day and time would be best. Bring the food in disposable
containers, so your friend won't have to worry about washing
dishes. Spend time sharing a meal.

- Go for a walk or outing together, but ask about and know your friend's limitations.

- Offer to help answer any correspondence that may be giving some difficulty or that your friend is avoiding.

- Call your friend and find out if anything is needed from the store. Ask for a shopping list and make a "special delivery" to your friend's home.

- Celebrate holidays and life with your friend by offering to decorate the home or hospital room. Bring flowers or other special treasures. Include your friend in your holiday festivities. A holiday doesn't have to be marked on a calendar; you can make every day a holiday.

- Check in with your friend's spouse, lover, care-partner, roommate, or family member. Though your friend is the one who is sick, they may also be suffering. They may also need a break from the illness from time to time. Offer to stay with the person with AIDS in order to give the loved ones some free time. Invite them out. Offer to accompany them places. Remember, they may need someone to talk with as well.

- Be creative. Bring books, periodicals, taped music, a poster for the wall, home-baked cookies, or delicacies to share. All of these become especially important now.

- Don't be reluctant to ask about the illness, but be sensitive to whether your friend wants to discuss it. You can find out by asking, "Would you like to talk about how you're feeling?" However, don't pressure.

- You don't always have to talk. It's okay to sit together silently reading, listening to music, watching television, holding hands. Much can be expressed without words.

- Tell your friend how good he looks, but only if it is realistic. If your friend's appearance has changed, don't ignore it. Be gentle; yet remember . . . never lie.

- Encourage your friend to make decisions. Illness can cause a loss of control over many aspects of life. Don't deny her a chance to make decisions, no matter how simple or silly they may seem to you.

• Be prepared for your friend to get angry with you for "no obvious reason," although you've been there and done everything you could. Permit this, and don't take it personally. Remember, anger and frustration are often taken out on the people most loved because it's safe and will be understood.

• Gossip can be healthy. Keep your friend up to date on mutual friends and other common interests. He may be tired of talking about symptoms, doctors, and treatments. Take your cues from your friend.

• What's in the news? Discuss current events. Help keep your friend from feeling that the world is passing by.

• Offer to do household chores, perhaps taking out the laundry, washing dishes, watering plants, feeding and walking pets. This may be appreciated more than you realize. However, don't do what she wants to and can still do for herself. Ask before doing anything.

• Send a card that says simply, "I care!"

• If you and your friend are religious, ask if you could pray together. Don't be hesitant to share your faith. Spirituality can be very important at this time.

• Don't lecture or direct your anger at your friend if she seems to be handling the illness in a way that *you* think is inappropriate. Your friend may not be where *you* expect or need her to be. You may not understand what the feelings are and why certain choices are being made.

• If you and your friend are going to engage in sex, be informed about the precautions that make sex safer for both of you. Heed them! Be imaginative . . . touch, stroke, massage. Sex need not always be genital to be fun.

• Do not confuse acceptance of the illness with defeat. This acceptance may free your friend and provide a sense of his own power.

• Don't allow the person with AIDS or her care-partner to become isolated. Let them know about the support groups and other concrete, practical services offered without charge by a local hospital or AIDS service-provider agency.

• Talk with your friend about the future: tomorrow, next week, next year. It's good to look toward the future without denying the reality of today. Hope is important at this time.

• Bring a positive attitude. It's catching.

• Finally, take care of yourself! Recognize your own emotions and honor them. Share your grief, anger, feelings of helplessness, or whatever is coming up for you, either individually with friends and loved ones or in a support group. Getting the support you need during this crisis will help you to be the real friend for your friend.

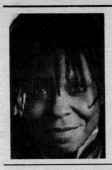

Whoopi Goldberg
THINK CREATIVELY!

Whoopi Goldberg began her acting career at age eight, when she joined the Helena Rubenstein Children's Theater. Her one-woman Broadway show, Whoopi Goldberg, *opened on Broadway in 1984.*

THIS BOOK HAS A LOT OF IDEAS about fighting AIDS. But don't let yourself be limited by the ideas that you read about here. There are things just waiting to be done, simply because no one has thought of them before. And there may be ways you can make a difference that aren't discussed here, because they depend on your unique skills or abilities. Ask a few questions of yourself:

What special skills do you have? If you're a carpenter, you could build a ramp that would allow more mobility for someone in a wheelchair. A good cook could provide hot meals for someone living nearby.

What can you teach? Michael Connolly of Boston's AIDS Action Committee tells of a young woman with cerebral palsy who strengthened her muscles through dance and movement classes. She now offers a dance therapy class for people with AIDS. A piano teacher in Florida offers free lessons to PWAs who have lost their eyesight.

How can you take advantage of what may seem like limitations? If you're housebound, you could offer much-needed babysitting services for a volunteer who's providing other services, or for a person with AIDS who needs a break from the demands of childrearing.

What can you offer? If you have a car, you can offer transportation to and from the doctor for someone without reliable transportation.

Are you overlooking the value of your personal presence? At Bellevue Hospital in New York, the AIDS Resource Center offers a visitation program with activities like reading or playing chess. There may be such a program where you live. Another need is for visitors in the home. Berit Pratt, AIDS Nurse Coordinator for the Visiting Nurse Association of Boston, stresses that their nurses can't always stay at a patient's home as long as they need to. Intravenous medicine, for example, can take five or six hours to administer, and the nurse must move on long before it's finished. With a minimum of training, a visitor can monitor this process, while helping the PWA deal with situations that might arise around the house while they're hooked up.

If you're ready to get involved in one of these ways, how can you hook up with the right people? Most larger cities have some sort of AIDS service organization that will guide you. But if that's not the case, then here's another need that should be met. Perhaps your first project should be to start some kind of similar coordinating network. With only a telephone and some volunteer help, you could at least begin providing a service to connect people who can offer services or help with those who would benefit from that help. The National AIDS Network (see the last chapter of this book) can provide advice.

3

AT HOME

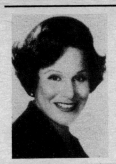

Abigail Van Buren

AN OPEN LETTER TO PARENTS

As the author for three decades of the "Dear Abby" column, Abigail Van Buren has become a household name. Her column is syndicated in over twelve hundred newspapers and has over ninety million readers.

DEAR PARENTS,

Those of you who have read my column during the past thirty years know that I have always urged open and honest communication between parents and children. My husband and I always made ourselves available to answer, to the best of our ability, any questions at any time. Some of the questions that came out of the blue were whoppers, and we often had family conferences if the subjects concerned "our family's" attitudes. "Family discussions" are an excellent tool for clearing the air, and we made a point of asking our children for *their* input, and we showed respect for their opinions. But the underlying message was always loud and clear: For an honest answer to any question, come to Mom and Dad. The door is always open.

But enough about my family and on to yours. Children should be told the facts of life as soon as they ask questions concerning the subject. Certainly, no child over the age of ten should be kept in ignorance "for his own good." For parents who cannot bring themselves to discuss anything relating to sex, there are books written by experts that will state the facts in language the child can understand. The school nurse may be a resource. The family doctor can help. But even if the parents can't do the talking, he or she should *be there* so the topic isn't separate from Mom and Dad.

And now, about AIDS . . . Call a family conference and ask your children what they know about AIDS. Listen carefully and correct any misinformation. Then offer these facts: People can become infected with this virus and show no symptoms for years — and yet, once they are infected, they can pass it on to everyone with whom they have intimate sexual contact.

Because there is no known cure for AIDS, there has been much panic and misinformation about how it might be spread. According to the American Foundation for AIDS Research, the best way to avoid getting AIDS is to never have unprotected sexual contact with anyone who could be infected, and to never share needles or syringes with another person.

Okay — so what is "unprotected sex"? In one sentence: unprotected sex is sexual intercourse without the use of a latex rubber condom *and* a spermicide containing the ingredient nonoxynol-9, which kills both sperm and the AIDS virus.

Can AIDS be caught from kissing? Or from sharing an eating utensil with someone who has it, or from being in a class with a student who has it, or from a mosquito bite, or eating in a restaurant that employs a person with AIDS? THERE HAS BEEN NO RECORDED CASE, TO DATE!!

But, back to basics. How can a boy, girl, man, or woman be certain that that potential sexual partner has never been infected with the virus, and therefore they are not risking their lives by having unprotected sex with someone "very special"? If I were talking to my child, I would stress that it is wise to wait until marriage to have sex — because the only 100-percent sure way not to get a sexually transmitted disease is to refrain from having sex. But, if they are already sexually active, or becoming sexually active, then they *must* know how to protect themselves and their partners.

Don't postpone talking to your children about AIDS. *Ex-*

plaining does not mean *condoning*. Children become sexually active earlier today than they did even twenty years ago. Parents will never reverse that trend by keeping children ignorant. Agreed, information about AIDS may take much of the "romance" out of sex. But it's up to you to start an ongoing dialogue with your pre-adolescents and teach them to understand the feelings they're experiencing as their bodies change and their hormones rage. What children don't know *can* hurt them.

So, Dear Parents, you are the front line of defense. If I can help further — that's what I'm here for.

Also a parent,
Abigail Van Buren

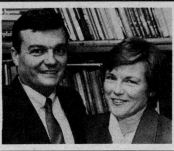

Ronald and Ann Moglia
TALKING TO YOUR CHILDREN

Ronald J. Moglia is the director of the Human Sexuality Program in the Department of Health Education at New York University. Ann Moglia is a counseling psychologist with a nursing background, and the former executive director of the Sex Information and Education Council of the U.S.

TODAY, MANY PARENTS ARE CONCERNED about how to talk to their children about AIDS. What your child learns now will lay a very important foundation for good self-esteem and health in the future. Here are some typical questions from parents:

At what age is it appropriate to begin telling children about AIDS?

Start when children have the ability to understand abstract ideas like viruses and communicable diseases, i.e., about third grade. Unfortunately, few children will wait that long before they ask a question about AIDS. In today's world they have probably heard the word and have sensed the fear around it long before that age. The parents of a child of any age should talk about AIDS as soon as the child has asked a question.

What is the first thing to say to children if they ask about AIDS?

The first thing is to be careful about your physical and emotional reaction to the question. Your reaction should be no different to this question than to a question about why the sky is blue. A shocked reaction to AIDS questions can discourage your child from asking more questions in the future. Second, *always* ask your child what she or he already knows about AIDS. The answer will give you invaluable insight about how to respond to what is of real concern.

What information should young children (five to eight years) be given about AIDS?

At this age, a child's understanding of the world is based on everyday life experiences. Therefore, your answers to questions should be based on concrete examples from your child's life. For example, if your daughter cuts her finger, this is a good time to explain how a virus (something that makes you sick) can get into the body through the blood system. Children this age also need to know that they are *not* going to get AIDS from friends or from things like cuts, nosebleeds, sharing gum, or mosquitoes.

What about pre-teens (nine to twelve years old)?

Children this age are experiencing the physical, emotional, and social changes of puberty. They are primarily concerned about their bodies, appearance, and what is normal. Some will start dating. It may also be the start of early sexual experiences and experimenting with drugs.

Because of the strong peer pressures that begin at this age, it is important that you discuss information about AIDS, regardless of what you know about your children's own sexual experimentation. Basic information about how AIDS is spread and how to be safe is essential for this age group. Doing this may seem like a difficult task, but it will give you a chance to teach your children the values you hope they will accept and adopt in their own lives.

What if my child doesn't ask any questions about AIDS?

Then bring the subject up. Do you wait for your children to ask if they can play with the stove?

You might begin by saying: "There is so much discussion

about AIDS these days. What kinds of things have you been hearing about it?" Starting a discussion after a TV show on AIDS or using a newspaper or magazine article can also open the door for discussion. Don't be discouraged if your child is not interested or comfortable talking at first. By bringing the subject up, you have let him or her know that you are open to future discussions.

I haven't talked about sexuality in general with my child. I don't feel very comfortable talking about AIDS. What can I do?

It's never too late to let your children know that you want them to have good information and help in understanding their developing sexuality in this age of AIDS. You, as a parent, have a wonderful opportunity to help your child separate the horrible consequences of AIDS from the positive joys of human sexuality. When you talk with your children about sexuality and AIDS, you are also saying that you care about their health and happiness. This can be one of the greatest joys of parenting. You can even tell your child that you have no training in this, but that you think it's important for you both to know all you can about AIDS. The family can learn about AIDS together!

Many parents have this concern because it is difficult to talk about something if you do not feel comfortable or prepared. Schools, religious groups, and community agencies have written materials available for parents that can be helpful.

What information should teenagers be given about AIDS?

Teenagers are learning to be more independent from their families. This is why friends and the peer group are so important. Social pressure to "fit in" is strong. Physically, teens are experiencing adult sexual feelings and desires. They are also trying to understand their sexual identity and values. Because of all these changes and choices, it is easy to see why interest and pressure to try sexual behaviors or to experiment with drugs can be very strong.

Although many parents are not aware of their children's

experiences, research reports indicate that the majority of teens in the United States experiment with drugs and sexual behaviors before they graduate from high school. Because these behaviors are *high risk* for getting AIDS, it is *essential* that *all* teens have detailed, candid, and accurate information about how to reduce the risk of getting AIDS.

How can I talk about safe sex or anal intercourse with my adolescent son or daughter?

Talking about sexual matters is not easy when you have not had much experience. Most parents feel this way. Your son or daughter does too! As a parent, it's up to you to take the first step, break the ice, and say: "I want to talk with you about AIDS. I want you to have answers to your questions and to know how to protect yourself." Once you've done that, you have opened the doors and have let your child know that you care and want to help. Remember, your teen is the expert in the family about your community's teen culture. Use that expertise to open communication with your child. For example, you might ask: "What are your friends saying about AIDS?"

I know my teen is not sexually active or using drugs. Why should I talk about AIDS?

This is the *best* time to talk about AIDS! Preventive education is the only defense against this disease. Equally important, talking about AIDS can alleviate anxiety that many young people now have about getting AIDS. Often these fears are focused around misinformation such as getting AIDS through swimming.

How can I talk about AIDS with my teenager and still have sexuality be something that is positive and wonderful?

Never before have parents been faced with such a responsibility to help their children grow up sexually. Many parents fear that sharing this information with their teens will remove the romance, the beauty, and the joy of healthy adult sexuality.

This is because most parents had little experience with sex education in their own growing-up experiences. In truth, learning the facts of sexuality only decreases ignorance and myths and enhances respect for the beauty, responsibility, and very special joys of being male or female.

RESOURCES:

• *How to Talk to Your Children About AIDS*. Single copies of this pamphlet are free; send a self-addressed, business-size stamped envelope to SIECUS/NYU Brochure, 32 Washington Place, Suite 52, New York, NY 10003. Prices for bulk copies are available on request.

• *AIDS and the Education of Our Children: A guide for parents and teachers*, published by the U.S. Department of Education. Single copies are free from the Consumer Information Center, Dept. ED, Pueblo, CO 81009.

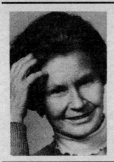

Elizabeth Winship
TALKING TO YOUR PARENTS ABOUT AIDS

Elizabeth Winship writes the nationally syndicated "Ask Beth" column for teenagers and their parents. She has written three books: Ask Beth: You Can't Ask Your Mother; Reaching Your Teenager; *and* Human Sexuality, *a textbook for high school students.*

DO YOU WISH YOU COULD TALK to your parents about AIDS? It would be a comfort to be able to share your ideas and your worries with the people who love you best. But AIDS involves sex and drugs and death — three things parents and teens have the hardest time talking about.

How can I bring the subject up without freaking them out?

Talk to them separately, some quiet time when you're feeling pleasant towards each other. Start with the less controversial aspects, for instance: "Dad, I heard AIDS has a long incubation period. What does that mean?" or "Mom, some people say everyone should be tested for AIDS. Do you think so?" Once you have broken the ice, you can go back to them for answers to vital questions like: How do you get AIDS? Is it safe to kiss people? Can you get it from toilets?

Suppose they say, "Why do you want to talk about that? Kids don't get AIDS!"

Tell them not many teens — less than two hundred — are

AIDS patients now, but thousands of people in their twenties have it. Many of them must have become infected in their teens since it takes up to ten years or more for the illness to show up. Many teenagers do have sex or use drugs, so you're scared. You need answers to questions so you can be sure how to protect yourself.

How could I talk about the gross stuff like condoms or intercourse or IV drugs?

Don't bring it up until you are discussing easier topics successfully. Then say you're embarrassed, too, but you can't talk about AIDS without including these subjects. Mentioning an outside source like your school, TV, radio, or a newspaper will make the issue sound impersonal, less likely to be connected to you personally.

Suppose they accuse me of having sex or using drugs?

You could say AIDS is something everyone needs to know about, in order to stay healthy. If you *have* had sex or used drugs, be honest if you can, and if you decide this admission will do good, not harm.

Suppose my parents think I'm asking because I'm gay? And I am?

Say you've heard that AIDS is not a "gay disease." It's being spread by IV-drug use and through sex with IV-drug users, to both men and women, too. So everyone needs to get the right information so they can avoid getting it.

Coming out to parents is a tremendously complex issue. Some parents can accept it, some can't. Don't do it without first talking with a knowledgeable and sensitive counselor.

Suppose my parents assume I'm asking because there's a kid with AIDS in our school?

This makes a good opportunity to discuss how AIDS is transmitted. Did you know there has been *no* known case of a person getting infected through casual contact, the kind kids have with each other every day at school?

I worry sometimes about dying from AIDS. How could I ever talk to my parents about death?

We're all afraid to talk about it because nobody really knows what happens after you die. Talk about something you've read or heard, or ask a direct question: "Are you ever afraid of dying?" or "What do you think would be the worst way to die?"

Suppose they get mad at me for asking about AIDS?

Apologize for surprising or shocking them, but say you worry about it and assume they do too. Then try again another day.

If it just can't work, or they hold it against you, find another trustworthy adult you can talk to, like another relative, a teacher, a counselor, or a doctor. A health professional would have information and wouldn't make emotional judgments about your asking.

RELATED READING:

• *AIDS: Questions and Answers*. Planned Parenthood Federation of America, 810 Seventh Ave., New York, NY 10019, or from your local chapter.
• *Coming Out to Your Parents*. Pamphlet available from Parents FLAG, P.O. Box 15711, Philadelphia, PA 19103.
• *The Kids' Book About Death and Dying*, by Eric E. Rofes and students at the Fayerweather Street School.
• *Tiger Eyes*, by Judy Blume. A novel about the death of a friend.
• *Your Child and AIDS*. Available from the San Francisco AIDS Foundation, 333 Valencia St., San Francisco, CA 94103. Include a 6-by-9-inch envelope with 45 cents postage.

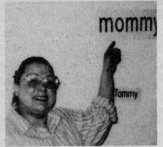

Eileen DeLamadrid

CHILDREN WITH AIDS NEED LOVE, TOO

Mrs. Eileen Gil DeLamadrid lives in New York City with Mikey and Johnny. She is a foster parent in the Leake and Watts specialized AIDS foster-home project.

TWO YEARS AGO I saw a newspaper story about children who had been born with AIDS. It showed pictures of the kids, and my heart went out to them. The only home these kids had ever known was a hospital room, because nobody wanted them. So I called the Leake and Watts Children's Home, which was mentioned in the story, and talked to Phyllis Gurdin who handles their foster-care program for children with AIDS and who turned out to be a wonderful person. Within two months, I had visited three-year-old Mikey in the hospital, and soon after that, I brought him home. When he came into my home, that was the first time he'd ever lived anywhere except in a hospital.

I'll be honest. The last two years have sometimes been very difficult. When I first got Mikey, it was like getting a stray dog. He had a lot of anger and confusion inside him, and a lot of hatred and animosity toward other people. That didn't change overnight. It's taken love and understanding and a great deal of patience. But it's rewarding, because I can see the results.

Mikey is five now. He's a bouncy boy, full of energy. He was born already infected with the AIDS virus, and today he has full-blown AIDS. But that doesn't keep him from being a regular little boy who likes to play and talk and have fun. Since coming here he's had the usual colds and fevers, but he hasn't been hospitalized.

A year ago, Phyllis called and asked if I wanted another child. "Fine!" I said. "Bring ten if you want!" That's how I got Johnny.

Johnny was thirteen months old then. Like Mikey, he had been in the hospital since he was born. Johnny had the virus when he came to me. But about thirty percent of the kids who are born with AIDS seem to sero-convert — that is, the body fights off the virus. Johnny has been one of the lucky ones; he now tests negative for the AIDS virus.

Johnny's a little delayed in his learning. He's two years old now, but he acts more like an infant. It may have something to do with the virus, or just with spending the first year of his life in the hospital. But with time and love, I think he'll grow up to be a healthy little boy.

When I got Mikey, Phyllis went over the precautions with me for his care. For the most part, I do the same things I did before — I disinfect the toilet, I keep the house clean. It's just that now I'm taking a few more precautions. The only precautions I have to use for myself are to use gloves when changing diapers, or when the children bleed. My main concern is for the boys. If I have a cold, I have to be careful not to give it to them.

The boys fill my day. They wake up very early: Mikey at around five, Johnny about five-thirty. Mikey loves to take baths in the morning. At eight o'clock, a bus comes to pick him up for day care. There are other kids with AIDS there, and it's been good for him. When he gets home he watches cartoons, or we read, or sing. We play together a lot.

Johnny's here all day, and he keeps me busy. He likes to play too, and I take him out to the park, or we walk around visiting friends and getting together with other children.

These kids bring so much happiness to my home. I give them something, and they give me back more. The only low point comes sometimes when I put them to bed. I'll see them there asleep, and occasionally I wonder, *Are they both going to be here next week?*

One thing that helps is that foster parents get a check each month to help with the expenses we face. So there's no financial hardship. The boys get all their medical care through the foster-care agency. The agency is always there to help when we need it.

Sometimes I forget about the AIDS thing with these children, just like I forget that Mikey is black and Johnny is white and I'm Puerto Rican. They're children. We're a family. If they get sick, I'll deal with that. But in the meantime, they're normal, healthy, lively kids.

What *does* bother me is that there are still children for whom a hospital room is the closest thing they've ever known to a home. About a thousand children are expected to be born with AIDS this year *in New York alone.* And the numbers are getting bigger in other cities. I hate to think that any of those kids may have to live without knowing the love of a real family like ours. If enough of us pitch in, none of them will have to.

BECOMING A FOSTER PARENT:

In the New York City area, for more information, call Phyllis Gurdin at 914-376-0106. Or write the AIDS Specialized Foster Homes at the Leake and Watts Children's Home at 487 S. Broadway, Suite 201, Yonkers, New York, NY 10705. In other areas, if you'd like to consider becoming a foster parent to a child with AIDS, ask a social worker, a member of the clergy, or an adoption agency for guidance.

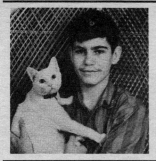

Ryan James

THE PET PALS PROGRAM

Ryan James wrote this as a thirteen-year-old, eighth-grade student at John Adams Middle School in Grand Prairie, Texas. He is an Eagle Scout Candidate. His mother, Ellen James, is the assistant head nurse at Parkland Memorial Hospital, and helped with this chapter.

I WANTED TO DO SOMETHING about AIDS but, as a teenager, I found my resources were limited. Therefore I decided to combine my interest in caring for animals and my desire to help people with AIDS. I became involved in a program to care for the pets of people with AIDS (PWAs) because I believe animals are great support for people who are sick or handicapped.

The first thing I did was to contact the AIDS Resource Center in Dallas. They suggested I go through the Volunteer Training Program. There I met other people who had been doing some work with animals, such as walking dogs or finding new homes for pets of PWAs who had become too ill to care for them. We decided to work together and we founded Pet Pals.

At first, Pet Pals was just a few people. We helped with vaccinations, feeding and grooming animals, and whatever else was necessary. We provided information, practical support, and financial assistance to PWAs so they could keep their pets at home with them. We also helped to clear up the misconceptions and fear about germs that pets may carry. Cats can carry CMV and toxoplasmosis, so people with AIDS need to be careful if they have cats as pets. Humans cannot give AIDS to pets.

I tried to think of ways to raise money, asking for donations and coupons for pet products and for grooming pets. Then a few veterinarians got involved, testing the pets and giving shots at a low cost. The Dallas ASPCA responded by donating time to help with heartworm testing.

Now enough people are involved for us to have one volunteer assigned to each pet. We're thinking creatively about other things to do: We've planned a Dog Show, and we even had a birthday party for a dog.

I have spoken to a group of people at the AIDS Resource Center about Pet Pals. At first it made me nervous, but the people were very supportive. It made me feel great when they came up afterwards to thank me. Several people said they had heard of Pet Pals but they did not realize someone thirteen years old had helped start it.

Ron Holder, who is Whoopi Goldberg's manager, suggested we could raise money by having a "celebrity auction" of autographed items. I've written to a few famous people, and they have mailed me things. People have been very generous, but we still need more celebrity items. So, if you have items you'd like to donate, please mail them to Pet Pals.

One fundraising idea I had was making a Haunted House at Halloween, but I didn't have a house to haunt and I couldn't do it by myself. So I asked if we could do it with other groups from the AIDS Resource Center and divide the work and funds. Adults and teenagers worked together on it. Although the Haunted House stayed open too late on school nights for me to help, I did work on the weekend.

This program was started as part of my Eagle Scout Community Service Project. That project calls for a Scout to plan, develop, and give leadership to others in a service project helpful to the community, and to think creatively of ways to raise money. As a Patrol Leader, I organized my troop to collect cans and newspapers.

I am the youngest founding member of the Pet Pals and my contributions are different from the adults'. Right now, my peers are entering the highest risk group. Our only defense against this deadly disease is education, which should start at an early age. Our fears keep us from believing that this can happen to someone we know. We need education, to learn that we have nothing to fear about casual contact with PWAs or their pets.

For many teenagers, AIDS is something very distant, something to be ignored, or perhaps joked about. My friends now know someone who sees people with AIDS regularly, and I think that makes it seem less mysterious to them. People occasionally ask about the Pet Pals program, and I think it's good for them to have a chance to talk about AIDS and to learn that people with AIDS have the same worries about their pets that anyone else would.

I feel that Pet Pals has been very successful and rewarding. The project is still in its infancy, and I would like to hear from other people who might be interested in working with pets of PWAs. There is much more that can be done. With each project we do, we think of ways to improve it for the next time. We expect Pet Pals to GROW!

FOLLOW-UP:

The Dallas AIDS Resource Center has information about starting a Pet Pals program. It's available from them at P. O. Box 190712, Dallas, TX 75219; 214-521-5124. Pet Pals can be reached at the same address.

4

IN SCHOOL
AND CHURCH

Timothy Arrison, Amy Fish, Ann Keane,
Jeff Lavin, Joanne Lavin, Margaret Pilaro,
Roxie Schroeder, and James Zezza

WHAT A HIGH SCHOOL CLASS CAN DO

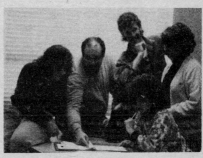

This chapter was written by Mr. Jeff Lavin's social studies class at Springfield High School, Springfield, Vermont.

THE HIGH SCHOOL CLASSROOM — with energetic and courageous commitment — can be a major catalyst in the war against AIDS.

We are a group of rural Vermont high school students, most of us from conservative backgrounds. Working on the AIDS issue at our school meant breaking a barrier. AIDS — and more particularly, homosexuality — had always been a subject no one was willing to talk about in the classroom. The walls came tumbling down in an unlikely place, to be sure: a quiet Vermont town nestled in the Green Mountains.

Last winter our class viewed the film *The Times of Harvey Milk,* an award-winning documentary about the life and tragic assassination of one of the first openly gay public officials in U.S. history. Milk, a city supervisor in San Francisco, was murdered along with the mayor, George Moscone, in 1979. The film opened our eyes about being gay, and specifically about the relationship between homosexuality and politics. The project eventually led to a class visit by Representative Gerry

Studds (D-Mass.) and publisher Sasha Alyson, two men whose wit and integrity changed many of our views about homosexuals and raised the consciousness of many parents and citizens. An activity such as this — controversial in many communities, but not especially risky if handled with sensitivity — is an important first step in breaking down the irrational fears and misplaced stereotypes about gay people.

We think it is important to destroy the connotation of the word AIDS as it is often heard in high school students' language: a code word or derogatory label for homosexuality. Students should learn the term "acquired immune deficiency syndrome" (most high school students do not know what "AIDS" stands for), and understand it as a medical issue.

Once you have committed yourselves to taking action against AIDS, we suggest the following activities for you to implement as part of your overall program:

• Invite guest speakers who will discuss the issue of AIDS, both socially and medically, such as members of the gay community or health professionals.

• Invite a person living with AIDS, as close to the class's age group as possible, to discuss the disease, its social pressures, and its medical complications. In preparation for your guest's visit, educate yourselves and others in the school about the medical evidence concerning how AIDS is actually transmitted. Some students, teachers, or parents may spread fears that letting a person with AIDS come into the school is dangerous. Address and rebut that kind of hysteria directly.

• Make current material readily available to all students so they can learn the facts about AIDS (see resources below).

• Request your local U.S. representative or senator, or other public officials, to address the class on what government is (and is not) doing in the fight against AIDS. Question government officials on what still needs to be done. Urge government action in no uncertain terms.

• Have an AIDS Awareness Week, which could include films, lectures, discussions, or a play about persons living with

AIDS (and their friends and families).

 • AIDS information should be added to current health education classes when they cover drug use and sexual conduct. These classes should be straightforward about the use of condoms and clean needles.

 • Another way to deal with AIDS awareness is to have open group discussions as part of current events curricula. In a world full of ignorance, knowledge and exposure is our best weapon.

 • After you have completed a number of the above suggestions (and consciousness has been raised to the point at which students are ready to act), organize school activities that center around student activism in the political arena. These may include displays, marches, fundraisers, petitions, letters-to-the-editor, etc. Consider any exercise in political activism that heightens awareness for greater funding for AIDS research as well as greater compassion for persons living with the disease. Parent and community involvement is essential.

However ordinary in ability you may think yourselves to be, all it takes are students who are extraordinary in commitment and energy. If you think you are — as we in Springfield, Vermont, do — go for it! The potential for educating your peers, teachers, and parents is limitless. Demonstrate to your community that social responsibility begins in the classroom.

RESOURCES:

• *The Times of Harvey Milk*, by Robert Epstein and Richard Schmiechen. Also available on video, from Pacific Arts Video (phone 1-800-538-5856).

• *AIDS and Your World*, a thorough 64-page booklet from Scholastic, Inc., provides material that could be the basis for a curriculum of anything from one to four weeks. For information contact Scholastic, Inc., P.O. Box 7501, Jefferson City, MO 65102; 1-800-325-6149.

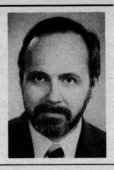

Stephen R. Sroka
WHAT TEACHERS CAN DO

Stephen R. Sroka is a teacher for the Cleveland Public Schools and the president of Health Education Consultants. He has trained over twenty thousand teachers.

SINCE EDUCATION IS OUR ONLY WEAPON in preventing AIDS, educators play a key role in fighting AIDS. Nearly 2.5 million teachers are teaching more than 47 million students across the nation. The teacher's role and influence is obvious, and here are some suggestions to help you educate our nation's youth about AIDS:

• *Don't reinvent the wheel.* Developing materials takes time and money. In the case of AIDS, time costs lives. Many existing materials (curricula, videos, pamphlets, etc.) can help you in your school-based AIDS-education efforts. Please see the suggestions at the end of this chapter.

• *Avoid AIDS education that is crisis-oriented and contributes to the AFRAIDS (Acute Fear Regarding AIDS) hysteria.* Put AIDS education into a sound education framework such as in a communicable-disease or family-health unit that can be taught as part of a K-12 comprehensive health education curriculum. This rational, conceptual approach helps to desensationalize and clarify the issues as well as allay the fears. It helps fight AFRAIDS.

• *Facts are not enough. Students need life skills taught early on.* Most programs are too biomedical. Knowing about T-4 helper cells is not enough to change behaviors.

We need programs to stress behavioral strategies to prevent AIDS, such as decision-making skills, assertive communication skills, stress-management skills, and self-esteem skills which empower our students to take control of their lives and practice health behaviors that reduce their risks.

These skills need to be introduced in lower elementary grades and stressed throughout the school years. As in advertising, to sell a product you must pitch it over and over. Just once in the ninth grade won't do it.

Avoid giving students conflicting messages. One group insists on teaching safer sex, another on teaching only abstinence.

We can no longer separate our AIDS-education efforts from others because of whatever differences may exist. Teachers must work with health departments, churches, parents, concerned agencies, the media, the total community. We must all work to give our students *age-appropriate, consistent, sensitive, and realistic* messages regarding AIDS. Their lives are too valuable to give them less.

RESOURCES:

• *AIDS and the Education of Our Children: A Guide for Parents and Teachers*, U.S. Department of Education. Send requests to: Consumer Information Center, Dept. ED, Pueblo, CO 81009.

• *Educator's Guide to AIDS and Other STD's*, Stephen R. Sroka, Health Education Consultants, 1284 Manor Park, Lakewood, OH 44107; 216-521-1766.

• *Guidelines for Effective School Health Education to Prevent the Spread of AIDS*, put out by the Centers for Disease Control, and available from National AIDS Information Clearinghouse, P.O. Box 6003, Rockville, MD 20850; 1-800-458-5231.

• National Association of Teachers of Comprehensive Health Education, 6020 Miles Avenue, Huntington Park, CA 90255; 213-582-4550.

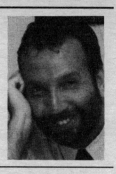

Eric E. Rofes
WORKING WITH YOUR LOCAL SCHOOL BOARD

Eric E. Rofes has taught sixth-grade classes in Cambridge, Massachusetts. He and his students have authored three books, including The Kids' Book of Divorce *and* The Kids' Book About Death and Dying. *He is now the executive director of Shanti Project in San Francisco and a member of the Los Angeles County Commission on AIDS.*

IN ATTEMPTING TO MOTIVATE SCHOOLS to play a useful role in our effort to stop AIDS in the United States, we have become convinced that local school boards and school committees have a critical function. Because of the controversial issues surrounding AIDS, it is often difficult for individual educators and school administrators to take the lead in facilitating an appropriate response from within their schools.

School boards are an efficient and far-reaching policy-setting body: their policies affect huge numbers of children, parents, and teachers. In AIDS prevention efforts, school boards can address two critical issues:

• Ensuring that good curricula are in place at all levels of schooling;

• Preventing panic and victimization by creating human policies surrounding HIV-infected students and staff members.

You can bring about positive changes in the lives of your local children and teenagers by urging the active support of your local school board in addressing these issues. Whether you are a student, a parent, or simply a concerned voter in the community, you have an interest in making sure that your city or town gets involved in this effort.

To motivate your school board and ensure appropriate and useful response, consider these possible actions:

• Arrange meetings with key members of your local school board and bring along two other community members. At these meetings, impress upon the school board members the need for establishing sound policies *before* your school district has to confront HIV-infected students or staff members, so that policy does not get formulated in emergency reaction to a new situation. Tell them why you believe it is critical for AIDS prevention information to be included in the schools' curriculum.

• Make a few phone calls and find out what other local school committees are doing. If they're doing nothing, approach yours, asking them to "take leadership" in the area on these issues. If others are already implementing policies or programs, ask for written information and pass this along to your school board. It's often easier for public officials to take action if they are aware that other school departments have already moved ahead on this issue.

• Organize a meeting of about a dozen local people who share your interest and commitment in doing something about AIDS. Have these friends and neighbors over to your home for a meeting and together make plans to lobby your school board, attend the next school board meeting (call ahead if you want to be placed on the agenda), or send a letter to the school board.

Be sure your school committee knows that they do not have to reinvent the wheel in terms of creating policies or developing curriculum. Over the past five or six years, many organizations, schools, and educators have taken the lead in developing materials that will be useful to you.

FOLLOW-UP:

For information about public policies in schools, contact Lambda Legal Defense and Education Fund, 666 Broadway,

New York City, NY 10012, 212-995-8585; National Gay Rights Advocates, 540 Castro Street, San Francisco, CA 94114, 415-863-3624; or the local affiliate of the American Civil Liberties Union. Educational materials and curricula can be found by consulting the local AIDS project in the nearest large city.

Sandra L. Caron

AIDS
ACTION
ON
CAMPUS

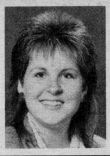

Sandra L. Caron is assistant professor of Human Sexuality and Family Relations at the University of Maine, and is co-chair of the National Coalition on AIDS and Families.

THE COLLEGE CAMPUS, with its highly mobile and sexually active adult population, provides many opportunities for AIDS to spread. Here are some ideas for preventing that spread.

• *Individual initiatives:* Educate yourself and share that knowledge. Be ready to dispel myths as you hear them arise. Force a person with a "fact" to cite the source; have sound information to back up your own position.

• *Get the message out:* Ask your campus newspaper to do an article or a series of articles about AIDS. Write letters to the editor. Contact your campus or local radio and television stations about airing public-service announcements about AIDS.

Design large posters or displays for areas both on campus, such as the student union, campus store, library, health service, and off campus, such as bars, restaurants, and laundromats. These could be developed by students majoring in art or advertising.

The educational messages should be simple (e.g., Ithaca College's "AIDS: Awareness Is Definitely Sexy"), and focus on the positive (e.g., the University of Maine's poster: "Are you playing the numbers game? Lower the risk of AIDS by using a condom and reducing the number of your sexual partners.").

Avoid negative messages like: "AIDS kills."

Use films and videos to educate. Ask the school health service to purchase films and videos such as *AIDS: Changing the Rules*. These short films can be shown alone or in conjunction with feature films shown on campus.

Distribute literature. Order free brochures from your state health department. They can be distributed at registration to all incoming staff and students, during sorority and fraternity rush, and at graduation.

Promote condom use. Talk to your campus paper about distributing condoms with an issue, as they did at Mansfield University in Pennsylvania. See that condoms are made available in the campus store, health service, or in vending machines around campus. Celebrate National Condom Week, February 13-19. Throughout the week run educational ads in the campus newspaper, give away "safer sex kits," and sell condomgrams (a condom with a Valentine's Day message).

• *Approach other campus groups:* Work with them to develop and disseminate information about AIDS both within and outside their organization. Gay and lesbian student union groups and health-related student groups are a good place to start.

Ask the campus programming board to sponsor speakers on campus. They could include someone from the local AIDS task force, an alumnus who now works with the issue, speakers from organizations like Gay Men's Health Crisis or the National AIDS Network, or authors of key books on AIDS. Speakers on related topics, specifically homophobia, are also important.

Talk to your library and campus bookstore about carrying a wide range of books and journals related to AIDS.

Urge the theater department to stage a production depicting the AIDS crisis or homophobia.

• *Get support from the administration:* Make an appointment with your college president, chancellor, or board of trustees. Work to develop a campus-wide task force on AIDS involving key administrators, faculty, staff, and students. This task force should develop the school's policy on AIDS, if one does not already exist, and offer support for educational efforts.

Request that the administration assign or hire a person to coordinate AIDS education on campus.

• *Peer education:* Urge your school to sponsor a Peer AIDS Education Program. This program should train a group of students to offer workshops on AIDS-related issues such as sexual decision-making, communication, and safer sex. Workshops can be held in residence halls, fraternities and sororities (make them mandatory for pledges), classes, and student unions. Develop a logo for visibility.

Organize an AIDS Awareness Week every semester. Peer educators can work with a number of campus and community groups to provide numerous educational activities.

Develop a campus AIDS resource guide. Peer educators can do the research. Make it available for students, staff, and faculty. It should state the campus policy on AIDS; list all services available on and off campus related to AIDS; and give information on library resources for students doing papers on AIDS-related topics.

FOLLOW-UP:

Write the American College Health Association, Richard P. Keeling, Chair of Task Force on AIDS, 1300 Piccard Drive, Suite 200, Rockville, MD 20850; 301-963-1100.

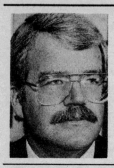

Representative George Miller

OTHER WAYS OF EDUCATING OUR CHILDREN

Congressman George Miller (D-Calif.) is chairman of the Select Committee on Children, Youth and Families, which published "A Generation in Jeopardy: Children and AIDS," a report on the effects of AIDS on the nation's children and teenagers.

THERE'S NO QUESTION that it's vitally important to educate our children about AIDS. Unfortunately, many parents feel acutely uncomfortable discussing sex with their children, so much so that they put it off indefinitely. Yet whether through formal coursework, family discussions, or other sources, we must educate our children about AIDS.

As a parent, I am acutely aware of the difficulties inherent in frank family discussions. As chairman of the Select Committee on Children, Youth and Families, I am also aware that AIDS poses a growing threat to the nation's young people. Today some 70% of girls and 80% of boys engage in sexual intercourse by age twenty. Teens who use no contraception or contraceptive methods other than condoms have no protection against AIDS. Yet only 15% of sexually active teenage girls report that their partner used a condom in their last sexual encounter. In a society where an estimated 21% of all AIDS patients were infected teenagers, we cannot allow our children to take these risks.

The AIDS epidemic is not going to go away, and failing to educate our children about it places them at increased risk. To date, only twenty-eight states require AIDS education in the schools. Fortunately, in our 1987 report on children and AIDS and subsequent investigations, the Select Committee found that many communities are responding creatively to the AIDS education gap. In Montgomery County, Maryland, for example, family-oriented programs include Teen and Family Conferences on AIDS held at churches, synagogues, and other locations; parent-teacher association AIDS Nights which offer education and dialogue for the entire family; and AIDS week at local high schools, where students are educated about different facets of the AIDS crisis for a few hours every day for a week. Similar programs could be set up in other communities through parent-teacher groups, scout troops, libraries, or religious organizations.

Where these education options are not available, parents who find it difficult to talk face-to-face to their children about AIDS should make sure the children talk with someone who *is* informed and comfortable with the issues. Here are a few suggestions:

• Identify adults who are well informed about AIDS and to whom your child feels close, such as the family doctor, the school health educator, local clergy, a relative or neighbor. Ask if they would be willing to discuss AIDS with your child.

• Find out whether the community groups such as the YMCA, scouts, 4-H, or special youth education and training projects have developed programs on AIDS. Tell your child about them.

• Get books, pamphlets, or videos from your Red Cross office, health department, doctor's office, or bookstore. For example, the Red Cross has developed an AIDS prevention program for young people; it includes a pamphlet with facts about AIDS, a video, and a parent-support brochure. The U.S. Public Health Service publishes *The AIDS Prevention Guide,* which includes numerous pamphlets and facts to help educate children and families about AIDS. The U.S. Public Health Service also sponsors a toll-free National AIDS Hotline (1-800-

342-AIDS) that can send additional written materials, as well as offering referrals to AIDS education groups and resources in your community. The Department of Health and Human Services has several brochures, including "AIDS Information for Young People." Use these resources and find out what else might be available.

• Take home the information you gather, review it yourself, and put it out where your child will see it. Try to identify someone to whom you can direct your child to answer questions and for further discussion.

• Find out if AIDS education is included in your local school's health curriculum. If not, work with local school groups to make sure such curricula are developed.

These few suggestions are but a start. Until we find a cure for AIDS, our children will live in a world where the disease poses a constant threat. We should regard providing education about AIDS as a crucial part of our children's upbringing, helping ensure them a healthy childhood and a safe, happy adulthood.

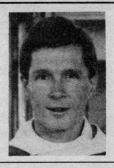

Zal Sherwood
HOW CONGREGATIONS RESPOND TO AIDS

Zal Sherwood is an Episcopal priest currently serving at St. Paul's Episcopal Church in Jackson, Michigan. He is the author of Kairos: Confessions of a Gay Priest.

RELIGIOUS COMMUNITIES CAN MAKE a valuable contribution to our society's response to AIDS no matter what their locality. The experience of many synagogues and parishes nationwide has proven that.

My parish, St. Paul's Episcopal Church in Jackson, Michigan, sponsors an active ministry to prisoners with AIDS. Teams of two parishioners take responsibility for visiting and caring for prisoners with AIDS at Jackson State Prison. In addition, at the request of a gay organization in Detroit, my parish has sponsored a safe-sex workshop for gay men. This was controversial — it was in fact picketed by fundamentalist church groups — but the congregation was very supportive. The fact that it could be done in Jackson, Michigan, shows that it could be done in most communities if the educational groundwork is done.

Trinity Episcopal Church in San Francisco has an extensive ministry to persons with AIDS, which includes feeding and housing PWAs within the parish. It also sponsors healing services every Sunday.

Roman Catholic and Episcopal dioceses and Presbyterian synods have founded hospices for persons with AIDS in New

York, New Jersey, Connecticut, the District of Columbia, Michigan, and California.

Chaplains from Christian and Jewish backgrounds are trained and employed full-time in pastoral care to persons with AIDS in New York, Miami, Chicago, Washington, San Francisco, and Los Angeles.

Educational resources on AIDS and spirituality have been developed by Roman Catholic, Episcopal, Presbyterian, Lutheran, and United Church of Christ denominations. Educational programs include sections on human sexuality, responsible sexual behavior, prejudice and homophobia, and religious response to pain, suffering, and mortality.

Many religious bodies have designated days of prayer for persons with AIDS and those who care for them. Churches and synagogues in most major U.S. cities have held services of prayer and healing for persons with AIDS.

But it's not only in larger cities that AIDS-related programs are happening. John Preston has told me of many examples in Portland, Maine, where he lives. The First Parish Society (Unitarian Universalist) of Portland donated space for the AIDS Support Group and other organizations as they were just forming, when rental fees could have been prohibitive. Holy Innocents (Roman Catholic) Church in South Portland has expanded its home-visitation program to include delivering meals and household help to people with AIDS.

The Episcopal Diocese of Maine has designated part of a priest's vocation to education about the disease in parishes throughout the state, making sure that the burden of spreading understanding about the human dimensions of AIDS doesn't fall solely on gay organizations, thereby helping to alleviate prejudice and ignorance about the disease.

As the largest city in Maine, Portland is the center of medical care in the state. Many patients receiving therapy there are far from their hometowns and families, and at least as many have been shunned by those very important people. Congregations in Portland have reached out to these individuals. These parishes and synagogues can become a surrogate community, giving support while the emotionally traumatic and physically difficult treatments are received in our hospitals.

These and other congregations' responses to people with AIDS offer the beginning models of how religious communities can respond to this crisis. The call of the congregation is to be a place where love and comfort are available to all, and especially to those unloved in the greater community. Church affirmation of the membership of PWAs in the personhood of all of us is the best of the church's message.

5

IN THE WORKPLACE

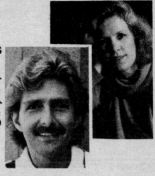

Dell Richards
WHEN A CO-WORKER HAS AIDS

Dell Richards is a freelance journalist whose syndicated profiles appear nationwide. The author of The Rape Journal, *Richards is currently working on a novel.*

AS A PERSON WITH AIDS, Paul Jasperson has faced many awkward moments. Sadly, some of his worst experiences have come at the hands of "healthy" individuals, those who view people with AIDS as lepers.

But he has learned to cope. And in the process, he has taught his friends and co-workers how to overcome their fear. As a result of his struggle, Jasperson developed a checklist of how to treat people with AIDS.

Jasperson, 36, a well-known Hollywood hairdresser, was diagnosed with AIDS in July 1986. He was still in good health and working a year and a half later. But when he first found out he had AIDS, he was faced with a dilemma. He wanted to tell people he had AIDS but his boss was afraid the salon where he worked would lose business if he did.

For a year, Jasperson didn't tell anyone. He felt dishonest and the cover-up didn't work. He had been hospitalized; people knew something was wrong. He knew they would eventually find out what.

"I didn't want people talking behind my back and wondering what was wrong with me," Jasperson said. "When I was diagnosed, I thought how horrible it would be if people were whispering about me. I wanted everyone to know so there was no question." For Jasperson, that meant telling his clients and co-workers the truth.

The worst obstacle Jasperson faced was the fear of death — people not wanting to face their own mortality. "I think a lot of people didn't want to see me going through what they thought AIDS was about — of seeing the deterioration and death," he said.

But Jasperson's health didn't deteriorate. Over time, he became a model of strength and courage for clients and co-workers alike.

"In the two years that I've had AIDS, my co-workers have begun to use me as an example," he said. "They look up to me because I'm doing so well."

Because of his personal experience with AIDS, Jasperson has a few suggestions about how he'd like co-workers to respond to his situation. His thoughts will be valuable for anyone who works with a person with AIDS.

Don't treat me with kid gloves. "At first, people were delicate around me," Jasperson said. "They were very careful about what they said to me. Now they know I can take things."

Don't monitor my health. "The most annoying thing is when people continually ask you how you are with that very concerned tone in their voice, asking if you're losing weight or gaining weight. If you get that ten times a day, it's enough to drive you crazy."

Have patience, especially if I'm not feeling well. "People with AIDS can go from feeling great to feeling miserable and thinking they're going to die within a period of five minutes — that happens to me three times a day. My co-workers may think I'm milking the illness or being overly dramatic, but I'm not."

Let me make my own decisions. "If I'm not well, let me sit down for a while or take a ten-minute break. Don't assume you know what I need and try to send me home. Let me decide."

Don't think you understand how I feel. "Unless you've been there, you can't know. It's wonderful to have compassion, but no one can understand what it's like."

Let me know you're willing to help. But don't assume I need help if I don't ask. "A good analogy is with someone who is handicapped. If other people constantly push the wheelchair without being asked, it makes the person feel more helpless. If the person needs it, they will ask for it. Try to treat the person as normally as possible."

Read about AIDS and ask questions. "People are less afraid if they know more. Become informed even if it means asking me questions about it. One subject I do know about is AIDS."

Don't make me into a token. "I'm a person who happens to have AIDS. But in my mind if *all* I am is a person with AIDS, that's going to make it pretty tough because I'm much more than that."

Lawrence H. Williford
DOES YOUR WORKPLACE POLICY COVER AIDS?

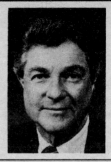

Lawrence H. Williford is vice president of corporate relations for Allstate Insurance Company, and a board member of the National Leadership Coalition on AIDS.

AN EARLY 1988 SURVEY sponsored by *Fortune* magazine and Allstate Insurance showed that America's top business executives believe AIDS is one of the country's most important problems — one that is likely to get even more serious in the future.

And they are correct. Because AIDS has such a major human and fiscal impact on American business, companies large and small must confront the question as soon as possible — preferably *before* an AIDS case actually arises within the workforce. Now and in the future, an AIDS policy is a must for every corporation.

But how should a company go about developing such a policy? What should it include? And what form should it take?

Representatives from more than two hundred major corporations met at a forum sponsored by Allstate Insurance to answer those questions. Their recommendations about developing policy with respect to AIDS in the workplace were compiled in a comprehensive report and presented to Secretary of Health and Human Services Otis Bowen in January 1988.

First of all, the report said the development of a company AIDS policy must have the active support of top management.

The policy itself should be created, and updated as necessary, by a task force that includes representatives from such areas as corporate communications, medical, employee relations and human resources, legal, safety, affirmative action, and corporate philanthropy. The task force should also include members from management and labor unions, where applicable.

In addition to these in-house resources, the group should call on outside experts in such areas as medicine and the law for guidance in policy development. The task force should analyze workplace risks with respect to individual businesses and geographic areas. It should consult with other employers and community groups to determine what kinds of policies have been adopted by other businesses and institutions.

And when all is said and done, the task force should develop a policy that maintains a safe work environment for all employees, while at the same time treating persons with AIDS with care and understanding. Specifically, the policy should:

- Provide a plan to educate employees, particularly with respect to how AIDS can be prevented. Emphasize that it is not transmitted through casual contact. Such efforts can help curb the spread of the disease, prevent panic responses among employees, and provide factual support for specific company policies with respect to AIDS in the workplace.

- Treat AIDS like any other life-threatening illness. Several court cases have established the precedent that AIDS is considered a handicap under state and federal law, and persons with AIDS are therefore entitled to protection from discrimination. AIDS cannot be used as a factor in hiring and firing decisions. Corporate policies should also allow affected employees to continue working as long as possible, provide reasonable accommodations and job modification where appropriate, and maintain eligibility for all company benefits;

- Discourage testing for the HIV virus within the employee population;

• Guarantee the confidentiality of all medical information related to AIDS;

• Provide for referral of affected employees to appropriate company and community resources and experts for consultation and treatment; and

• Encourage creative corporate philanthropy with respect to AIDS, especially in the areas of research, education, care and treatment, and technical assistance.

In short, corporate AIDS policies should be both consistent and compassionate. They should be tailored to the needs of individual companies. But above all, they should be developed soon — AIDS is an issue that cannot, and should not, be ignored any longer.

Alan Emery
TAKING SENSIBLE PRECAUTIONS ON THE JOB

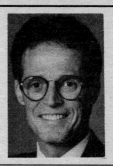

Alan Emery is a psychologist, management consultant, co-author of Managing AIDS in the Workplace, *and an international consultant on AIDS in the workplace.*

THE HIV EPIDEMIC provides the opportunity for all of us to review the sensible precautions we should be taking on the job as well as in our personal lives. HIV — the human immunodeficiency virus — is very hard to get. Yet even in workplaces where there are no risks of contracting HIV, there is often fear, confusion, myth, and misinformation about the disease. And that's where the dangers are.

HIV is not casually contagious. You cannot get HIV in the regular routine of the normal work environment. You cannot get AIDS from sharing the same desk, chair, typewriter, paper, pencil, computer, drinking fountain, cafeteria, elevator, toilet seat, or any other object in the workplace. In the conventional workplace you cannot contract HIV from routine interaction with your co-workers, even if a co-worker is infected with HIV.

Try to clarify what your concerns are, what you are not clear about, or what is it you don't really believe, and then ask questions. What about paper cuts? Is the cafeteria really safe? What do I do in an accident? Take your questions to the company nurse or your union representative or the human resources department. Tell them about your concerns and ask them to provide you and your co-workers with the information you need. Call the National AIDS Hotline (1-800-342-AIDS) for answers to your questions. Look up your state's AIDS hotline number and call them too. The hotlines have the answers you need. Contact your local AIDS organization, the Red Cross, and your local department of public health for brochures and materials. In the conventional workplace, taking sensible precautions on the job means getting all the information you need to feel safe.

As an employer, even if your workplace poses no risk of infection for HIV, find out what your employees' concerns and questions are. Then find ways to address their concerns and get answers to their questions. The Presidential Commission on the HIV epidemic identified discrimination as the most significant obstacle to progress against the epidemic. Be certain that your company and employees do not discriminate against people with HIV. Form an HIV committee to deal with policy development and employee education. Talk with your colleagues and your professional organizations and find out what they are doing. Contact the San Francisco AIDS Foundation for information on their AIDS-in-the-workplace programs. One contact will lead to another and you will quickly find the resources you need for your organization.

There are some occupations where specific precautions should be taken to avoid the possible transmission of HIV or any other disease. These occupations include police officer, firefighter, emergency worker, health-care worker, and other professions where direct contact with infected blood can occur. All of these occupations have policies and guidelines to avoid the spread of infectious diseases, including HIV. These guidelines are established by the Centers for Disease Control in Atlanta, as well as other regulating agencies. People in these occupations have always had risks of infection that people in other jobs have not had. For example, hepatitis-B is far more contagious than HIV, and can be deadly. Follow the guidelines for avoiding hepatitis B and you will also be protected from HIV.

Health-care employers and employees should follow the guidelines of the U.S. Public Health Service's "Recommendations for Prevention of HIV Transmission in Health Care Settings." The American Red Cross in Sacramento developed the "AIDS Education for Emergency Workers" project. This project provides materials and training that explain in detail the precautions police officers, firefighters, emergency medical technicians, probation officers, jail staff, and other emergency workers need to take on the job. Contact your professional association and ask for their recommendations. Review the guidelines and policies regularly.

All workers should be provided with HIV education and information so their understanding of the disease is clear, accurate, and up-to-date. Discrimination against people with HIV must stop. If you know the facts about the disease, follow the guidelines specific to your occupation, and don't engage in the behaviors that transmit the disease, then you are not going to get HIV.

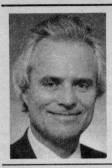

Bryan Lawton

SETTING THE TONE IN YOUR COMPANY

Bryan Lawton is Executive director of employee assistance services of Wells Fargo Bank in San Francisco, and serves on the board of the National Leadership Coalition on AIDS.

THE FEAR OF AIDS IN THE WORKPLACE is entirely natural, but we must be careful not to let that fear interfere with our judgment or our humanity. A carefully thought-out workplace policy is one step in this direction. But daily interactions create a tone within our companies that is just as important as an official written policy. And all of us, whatever our position, play a role in setting that tone.

When did you last hear — or tell — an AIDS joke in your workplace? If a co-worker is diagnosed with AIDS tomorrow, how do you think he or she will feel about coming back to work after hearing that same joke recently from a colleague?

If you're doing volunteer AIDS work, do you feel free to mention that fact to co-workers? Doing so will emphasize to them that AIDS is an issue that affects us all, and that all of us can do something about.

What kind of philanthropic and charitable-giving programs does your company have? There are many ways it could support AIDS work. If your firm has a matching-contributions program for certain non-profit groups, at least one AIDS organization should be on that list. Local AIDS organizations need a wide range of services and supplies; can your company make in-kind contributions of anything that would be useful? The initiative for this needn't come from the boss; there's no reason an employee can't make suggestions in this regard.

How is information disseminated in your workplace? Is there a bulletin board, or are memos frequently circulated, or is there a computerized bulletin board, or a company newsletter? That's an important place for AIDS information. If a misleading rumor about AIDS is circulating in the company, a well-documented notice on the bulletin board discussing the issue will not only help set the record straight — it will also emphasize that the company considers this issue to be a high priority.

What are the many ways that attitudes about AIDS are being shaped within your company? What can you do to most productively make a difference?

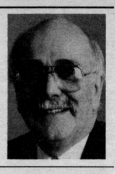

Bill Olwell
A UNION APPROACH TO AIDS IN THE WORKPLACE

Bill Olwell is executive vice president and international director of collective bargaining and negotiated benefits for the United Food and Commercial Workers International Union.

UNIONS HAVE A DUAL CONCERN of protecting the health of workers occupationally exposed to AIDS, and safeguarding the rights of workers infected with AIDS. Unions and management can work together to: (1) promote infection control, (2) accommodate workers with AIDS, (3) prevent discrimination, and (4) educate employees about AIDS.

Infection Control Programs: These programs seek to prevent worker exposure to all infectious diseases, including AIDS. All facilities where workers can come in contact with infectious diseases should develop such a program, including:

- guidelines that describe precautionary measures — for each occupation in the facility — to prevent the transmission of all infectious diseases, including AIDS;
- a worker-notification plan to inform all workers who could come in contact with infected blood of the hazard;
- protective equipment, provided by management, that enables workers to adequately follow the guidelines and protect themselves;
- a specific policy to respond to needlestick injuries and similar accidents;
- protection of client confidentiality.

Workplace Policies to Accommodate Workers with AIDS: Responsible workplace policies that accommodate workers with long-term illnesses, including AIDS, are critically needed. These policies should be implemented before an employee becomes ill, and should provide ill workers with the option of remaining at their jobs if they are not infectious. Unions and management should jointly develop workplace policies for AIDS and other long-term illnesses that:

- allow the worker and his or her physician to determine when and if the patient can continue working;
- allow alternative work schedules such as part-time work, short-term disability leave, and long-term disability leave;
- provide alternative work for someone who can still work but is unable to continue his or her particular job.

In addition, such policies must assure that no employee with AIDS faces discrimination. Workplace policies should contain specific provisions to:

- maintain the confidentiality of workers with long-term illnesses;
- continue to maintain health benefits or access to group coverage for sick employees;
- prohibit the use of antibody testing as a condition of employment, or any routine screening of employees, since AIDS is not transmissible through casual contact.

Worker Education and Training: Public concern about AIDS is understandable. Inadequate public education has resulted in a great deal of misinformation about the transmission of the AIDS virus. This has led to fear and panic, as well as to proposals for universal testing of workers in certain occupations (such as restaurant workers) even though there is no scientific justification for such drastic measures.

Worker education and training on AIDS should also be conducted. This training should be provided not only to workers who come into contact with the AIDS virus at work, but to all workers.

All employees should be provided with clear and accurate information regarding the transmission of AIDS. Workplace educational programs should be in place before an employee or co-worker becomes ill. A good program can go a long way toward alleviating unfounded fears should a co-worker become ill.

Federal Funding: Federal action on AIDS has been slow. A number of unions have called for increased federal funding to:
- develop guidelines to protect workers in all occupations from exposure to AIDS;
- conduct adequate research on the cause, transmission, prevention, and treatment of AIDS;
- provide medical and social support for AIDS-diagnosed persons and their families.

Father William J. Wood, S.J.
CLERGY HAVE A UNIQUE ROLE IN CONFRONTING AIDS

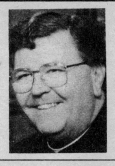

Father William J. Wood, S.J., is executive director of the state conference of Roman Catholic bishops in California; it was with his guidance that the California bishops published their landmark pastoral letter on AIDS, "A Call to Compassion," in the spring of 1987. He also serves as president of the Board of Trustees of the Institute for Food and Development Policy (Food First).

MEMBERS OF THE CLERGY of all religions are uniquely positioned to do something about AIDS. We enjoy access to congregations of ordinary people that no one else does. And we are generally trusted and respected by our flocks. Furthermore, clergy are specialists in proclaiming the Good News. If our society needs anything as much as trust and respect while we try to deal effectively with AIDS, it can only be the Good News of unconditional love and ultimate hope. That's what clergy have to offer by their very vocation.

More than a few of us have the privilege of ministering to persons with AIDS or of being otherwise directly involved in doing something about AIDS as a principal part of our assigned ministry. My younger Jesuit brother Jon Fuller, for example, cares for persons with AIDS at Boston City Hospital while he studies theology in preparation for ordination.

Almost as involved these days are still others — Jewish, Protestant, and Catholic clergy — who work as hospital chaplains. They not only minister to persons with AIDS but play a vital role in educating, sensitizing, and spiritually supporting the health professionals and staff of the hospitals.

Chaplains like John Healy of Mercy Hospital in Sacramento also give their energies to educating local communities outside the hospital about AIDS. And they are often part of teams that set up and promote home care and mobilize other community services for persons with AIDS. Such services also include counseling and support for those who test positive for HIV.

I am not the only member of the clergy whose principal ministry has to do with influencing public policy, particularly striving to provide a voice for the voiceless and most vulnerable in our society. High among my priorities is working for legislation that will effectively do something about AIDS — in terms of research, treatment, and prevention — while promoting the dignity and human and civil rights of persons with AIDS, AIDS-Related Complex, and HIV antibodies.

Most clergy do not have the opportunities I have just described as part of their ordinary ministerial work. But all clergy can exert a significant impact on AIDS in four ways that form part of the very fabric of their calling as God's ministers:

Pray — Listen to God's call: "The Spirit of the Lord is upon me, because the Lord has anointed me to bring good tidings to the afflicted; he has sent me to bind up the brokenhearted ... to give them a garland instead of ashes ... the mantle of praise instead of a faint spirit." (Isaiah 61:1-3)

Get to know people whose lives have been touched by AIDS: We may approach such people with a sense of giving and care, but the way they touch us and change us is an overwhelming experience. Mother Teresa talks about finding God in the people she serves. Archbishop John R. Quinn of San Francisco found his own life transformed and deepened by his intimate encounter with a person with AIDS.

Raise the consciousness of your congregation: Your people trust you. If you speak authentically from a profound prayer life and the experience of the world of AIDS, you will be able to allay their fears and raise them up to that perfect love that St. John tells us casts out all immobilizing fear.

Promote the formation of AIDS ministry teams: Encourage your people to study about AIDS in a way that leads to action. The traditional formula works: *observe, judge, act,* judging not people but what needs to be done and what can be done.

If every rabbi, priest, minister, and imam inspired one small group of people to do this, we would have a national campaign of unbelievable proportions!

FOLLOW-UP:

A wonderful sourcebook for religious professionals is entitled *AIDS: Spectre of Fear, Call for Concern: A collection of pastoral responses.* Copies can be obtained (for $5.00 postpaid) by writing Communication Ministry, Inc., P.O. Box 2272, Times Square Station, New York, NY 10108.

Joe Davidson

JOURNALISTS: GET THE STORY RIGHT

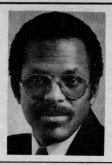

Joe Davidson is a reporter with the Wall Street Journal's *Washington Bureau and a lecturer in journalism at Howard University. He is a two-time Pulitzer Prize juror and a founding board member of the National Association of Black Journalists.*

ONE OF THE MOST unfortunate problems surrounding the AIDS crisis is the amount of misinformation it has generated. The epidemic is bad enough without adding uninformed, misleading, and just plain wrong information to the mix. Journalists are in a prime position to remedy that situation.

Journalists who cover the AIDS story must take special care to present the facts in a way that accurately portrays the urgency of the problem, but without exaggeration or sensationalism. New scientific developments, for example, may be worth reporting, but those stories should not lead to false hopes of an early cure or wonder drug when that remains a long way off.

The fight against the disease has been hampered by myths about how it's transmitted and who has it. Education is the single most important tool in that fight and journalists can be the best educators. We can run stories that specifically debunk notions such as calling AIDS a "gay disease."

Reporters may need educating and myth debunking before approaching the AIDS story in a fair and accurate way. People with AIDS, AIDS activists, and public-health officials can be invited to discussion sessions designed not only to provide information for print or broadcast, but also to shatter erroneous beliefs. We should not assume that generally well-informed journalists automatically escape bad information; *all* questions, no matter how elementary, should be encouraged at such sessions.

AIDS stories can come up on almost every beat. Look for them. Discuss interrelationships. Analyze coverage. What is the local government doing about the disease at public health clinics, for hospitals, and in the budget? What AIDS-related instruction is given police officers and firefighters; is it accurate? How has the business community responded? Have people with AIDS been unfairly treated by employers? Have customers with AIDS been unfairly treated by restaurants and clothiers? How are neighborhoods responding to facilities in their areas that deal directly with people with AIDS, or with drug treatment centers that are critical in the fight against AIDS? Do obituaries list AIDS as a cause of death? If not, why not?

Are there any local athletes with AIDS playing despite the disease? Are there any innovative AIDS-related projects in your area? Are churches taking an active interest in the epidemic? Are there good human-interest stories about AIDS workers? Are the highly opinionated columnists and talk show hosts conveying accurate information, or are they part of the problem?

Like many scientific issues, AIDS is complex. News desks and reporters should maintain contact with local experts who can be called upon to help evaluate information for background and on-the-record use. These experts can address journalism groups and discuss coverage and story ideas.

AIDS presents an opportunity to explore a variety of related health and socio-economic issues. For example, the relatively high incidence of AIDS within the black community points not to an immune deficiency problem peculiar to Afro-Americans, but to oppressive living conditions that too often encourage drug abuse, poor health, and little education. And the ability of the American health system to respond to the disease points to general shortcomings in such areas as long-term care.

Outside of work, there are also ways journalists can be a part of the solution. AIDS groups need public-relations advice in getting information to their constituencies. (Be careful not to violate any ethical standards. For example, don't write a press release for a group, then write a story based on that release.)

In the back of this book, you'll find information about organizations involved in AIDS work, and books that deal with the subject. Don't hesitate to get their advice any time you're unsure about the facts.

George Appleby

THE SPECIAL CHALLENGE FOR SOCIAL WORKERS

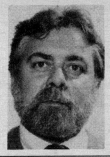

George Appleby, A.C.S.W., is a professor at Southern Connecticut State University School of Social Work and a member of the Governor's Task Force on AIDS.

THE TRADITIONS OF THE SOCIAL-WORK profession demand that we act on behalf of people in greatest need. The AIDS epidemic, more than any social problem in recent memory, tests our commitment to that principle.

Social workers have already taken the lead in many communities to form AIDS service programs. However, as professionals providing a wide array of health and human services, we are uniquely able to do much more. Specifically, we need to expand agency-based AIDS education, as well as AIDS-related health and social services.

Begin by suggesting that your agency study the in-service needs of staff and evaluate the need for agency-sponsored AIDS services. This plan should examine professional methods most effective in changing behavior that places a client at risk for AIDS.

You know that most people find it difficult to discuss sexual behavior and drug use. Most people have difficulty hearing information about safer sex or clean-needle use. These messages must be presented many times and in different ways. You can personalize information for each client, helping them think through and adopt new behaviors that are less risky. You can reinforce these personalized efforts by making written and video materials available in the agency's waiting room.

Encourage clients to use these same educational steps with friends and families. Your local AIDS project will have suggestions for materials designed for different groups. *Teaching AIDS,* by Quackenbush and Sargent, is a resource guide easily adapted to agency services.

The expansion of services should be based on a thorough understanding of what clients need. Your agency might find a need for self-help, treatment, and support-group services for persons with AIDS and their loved ones. Such groups should explore the progression of the illness, the impact of medications, non-medical treatment options, and legal and financial services. Bereavement groups are needed. Additional suggestions are presented in *Responding to AIDS: Psychosocial Initiatives,* edited by Leukefeld and Fimbres.

Drug-treatment programs, supervised housing, and skilled nursing-home and hospice care are needed in each community. Contact your local office of the National Association of Social Workers to see what is being planned and how you might get involved.

The need for service is great. No matter where or at what level you practice, your skills are needed. The first step is with your agency. After you have tackled that challenge, the volunteer programs in your community need your concern, your commitment, and your professional skill.

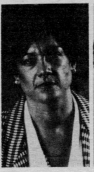
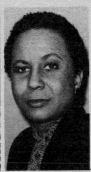

Jane Pinsky and Donna Rae Richardson

WHAT HEALTH WORKERS CAN DO

The authors are both on the staff of the American Nurses Association. Jane Pinsky is a lobbyist for civil rights issues, and Donna Rae Richardson has been a nurse for twenty years and a lawyer for twelve years.

THE AIDS EPIDEMIC HAS PRODUCED fear and anxiety among many health-care providers. This fear has triggered emotional and often irrational responses because many health-care providers do not know how the AIDS virus is transmitted and, more importantly, how it is not transmitted.

The American Nurses Association (ANA) was among the first health-care groups to address the issue of AIDS health care. ANA believes that all health-care providers should be educated about AIDS so they know what not to fear, and when and how to exercise appropriate precautions.

Precaution benefits both the health-care provider and the person with AIDS. The Centers for Disease Control recommends that a nurse or doctor wear gloves and sometimes a mask when examining or treating a person with AIDS. Some people believe this is to protect the health-care provider, but in fact, the person with AIDS, whose immune system is so vulnerable, needs the protection from infection as well. Since AIDS is transmitted mainly through the sharing of needles, semen-to-blood contact, or blood-to-blood contact, the AIDS patient is actually at a greater risk of catching a cold from a nurse or doctor than is the nurse or doctor of contracting the AIDS virus.

It is equally important for the health-care provider to explain the reasons for wearing protective garb to a patient and a patient's family, lover, or friends. Too often, people sense that the protective garb indicates that the virus can be transmitted by casual contact. This myth just adds to the all-too-prevalent confusion about how AIDS is and is not transmitted.

When the Department of Health and Human Services announced AIDS was the "number one health priority," ANA stated that all people who have AIDS have a right to equitable and humanistic health care, including: (a) quality treatment, including nursing and social support services, (b) non-discriminatory use of current isolation procedures, (c) full explanations of research procedures, treatment, and risks involved, (d) informed choice of treatment and research modalities, (e) confidentiality of the medical record, and (f) respect for privacy and significant relationships.

The ANA advocates that nurses treat AIDS patients with the same care and respect as they treat other patients. Keep in mind the importance of your role in caring for those who are ill. People with AIDS need affection like everyone else. Don't be afraid to touch someone with AIDS. You can't do that from a doorway; go into the patient's room and interact as part of your nursing-care plan. Try to get patients to verbalize their fears and those of the families and friends. AIDS is something everyone needs to talk about and understand. If nurses can be at peace with our understanding of the disease, we can be effective in our care and treatment of people with AIDS.

Health-care providers, especially nurses and doctors, have historically provided care to those afflicted with once-fatal infectious diseases, often at our own risk. We therefore have a certain amount of credibility about such illnesses. Now is the time to use that credibility and assume a front-line position in three areas of AIDS education.

Health-Care-Worker Education: All health-care workers should get a copy of the *Surgeon General's Report on AIDS* and the Centers for Disease Control's *Recommendations for Preventing Transmission of Infection with HIV Virus in the Workplace.* Those guidelines will protect you from hepatitis-B as well. Read them and share them with your family and co-workers. Do an inventory of your workplace to assure that the CDC Universal Precaution Guidelines are being followed. Demonstrate what is reasonable and what is not. Insist that your employer, for the benefit of worker and patient, do education and training on the disease and the precautions all health-care workers must follow. Work with professional groups to ensure the education and training of members. Advocate education for all levels of workers. Once you are knowledgeable, assume your responsibility to educate others.

Patient Education: More than ever, we must educate patients about AIDS. Such education must target those who have been infected with the virus, as well as non-infected patients, and it must include information about the disease and its prevention. Individual health counseling which addresses preventive health practices and the avoidance of high-risk behaviors must be provided by qualified health professionals.

Public Education: Health-care workers are neighbors, church members, students, parents, consumers, and community workers and are often consulted informally on health care issues. Use this opportunity to educate the public. When misinformation is presented by the media, respond with a correction in an editorial reply or letter. Offer to conduct education programs for church, PTA, school, and community organizations. Work with the Red Cross educational programs. Break the cycle of fear by providing factual information and setting an example for other health-care providers.

The health-care community must remain scientific, calm, and logical in our approach to AIDS. Oppose efforts to blame any group or nationality for this devastating disease. AIDS is an equal-opportunity disease; it affects all races, sexes, and ages. Speak out against discrimination and urge compassion. Most importantly, urge your public-health and other government executives to exercise leadership to ensure that education and health resources are available and accessible to all.

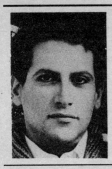

Harvey Fierstein
PEOPLE IN THE ARTS HAVE NO END OF CHOICES

Harvey Fierstein's Torch Song Trilogy *won the 1981 Tony Award for Best Play; two years later his* La Cage aux Folles *won the Tony for Best Musical. In 1989, Fierstein starred in the movie version of* Torch Song Trilogy.

REMAINING SILENT ABOUT AIDS is dangerous. Fear, frustration, anger, concern, and hope are but a few of the emotions that come to mind when I think about AIDS. These are not feelings that should be harbored unexpressed. What better way to open up, air, and share these strong feelings than through the arts? The essence of art is expression and communication. With art we can assure each other of our commonality and solidarity against this disease. Art also helps to replace heartless statistics with a human face and soul while educating and dispersing important information to the general public. Finally, the arts are a nifty way to raise money for the thousands of AIDS-related organizations struggling to provide necessary services in this crisis.

The Names Project is a San Francisco-based organization that is sewing together a giant quilt composed of individual memorial panels for people who have died with AIDS. You may have seen a display of this work in progress in the media. Why not create a panel for a friend or loved one? Information and specific requirements can be obtained from The Names Project; see Cleve Jones's chapter in this book.

Others in the visual arts can use their specific talents to create works that reflect their personal feelings about the AIDS crisis. Group showings of such work can be used as benefits, and the work itself can raise consciousness with each viewing. If you've the time to volunteer, perhaps you could contact a local organization and begin a workshop for people with AIDS. Helping others to express themselves in painting or drawing or other crafts is a gift of your time that will pay back a hundred-fold in satisfaction.

People in the performing arts field have no end of choices for their involvement. There are a great many plays and theater pieces already created concerning AIDS: Larry Kramer's *The Normal Heart*, *The AIDS Show*, and my own *Safe Sex*, to name a few. Why not get your local theater, university theater, or club to present one of these shows? Or if you've got the talent, create a show of your own. An AIDS benefit show need be no more than a local talent showcase. What's important is the concern, not the specific content. If you can't get the performers, but you know an auditorium that you can get your hands on, consider showing a vintage film or series of films to raise money. Once again, the words "AIDS benefit" will help raise consciousness and show that your heart is in the right place. If you're a singer, you can try contacting a local cabaret or bar or dinner theater about doing a benefit night. Poets and short story writers can have evenings of readings from their works, journalists can write and submit articles to local papers. . . . Whatever your field, whatever your talent, whatever your venue, the point is to show concern publicly about the AIDS crisis. When you show your concern, you free others to express theirs. Remaining silent about AIDS is dangerous. The arts can lead us to a safer world.

6

GOING FURTHER

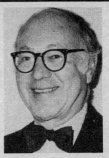

Ben Strohecker
THE
LEADERSHIP
IS YOU

Ben Strohecker has taken a one-year sabbatical from his position as chief executive officer of Harbor Sweets, a candy company in Salem, Mass., to raise funds nationwide for the care of people with AIDS through events called Aid & Comfort and to raise awareness of AIDS and HIV within small businesses.

TWELVE YEARS AGO, I started my own business. Once it was on its feet, I began to fantasize often about taking a year off for public service. I hoped to do this before I was too old to accomplish anything. Yet for many years, the day-to-day demands of the company made such a sabbatical seem like a distant fantasy indeed.

Then, in the spring of 1987, I learned about a San Francisco fundraiser involving the food and hospitality communities there. It was called Aid & Comfort, and it raised $400,000 for the care of people with AIDS. I realized then that the AIDS issue had been pulling me by the scruff of the neck. I wanted to get involved.

Fortunately, as a New England chapter board member of the American Institute of Wine and Food, I was in a position to do something. I worked with national AIWF chair K. Dun Gifford and several other board members to duplicate San Francisco's night of gourmet food and headline entertainment in Boston.

That was my first real opportunity to get involved in AIDS

fundraising. I coordinated activities, mediated problems, approached businesses for support, and tried to spread my enthusiasm to the 1000 (that's right, one thousand) volunteers who helped make it happen. All the food and beverages were donated and thirty-five of New England's leading chefs volunteered their time. We had no trouble selling tickets, and grossed $500,000 for the care of people with AIDS.

We also raised some consciousness. Aid & Comfort gave many segments of the population their first chance to become involved in this issue. Chief executive officers interacted for the first time with AIDS activists and people with AIDS.

By the time Aid & Comfort had ended, I was ready to move ahead with my fantasy of a taking a year off from my business to devote to public service. I had founded my company, Harbor Sweets, with the goal of making the best candies that were humanly possible. From the first test batch in my kitchen at home, the company grew to 150 employees. We had developed a proud record of hiring people some of whom are often considered "unemployable" — and found a way for each of them to become a productive member of our staff.

Now I needed to convince my employees, my management team, my bankers, and my directors that it was no longer a one-man show. The only way to do that was to leave for an extended period. My goal of taking a year off for public service coincided with the real needs of my business.

The challenge was to match my skills and experience to the needs of fighting AIDS. I soon realized that after my twelve years at Harbor Sweets, I could bring several valuable skills to this new arena.

My marketing experience could be helpful in getting corporate support and good turnouts for fundraisers. Harder to define, but equally important, I had experience in coordinating many distinct activities toward one final goal.

But most important, I could approach the business community as an insider. Most AIDS activists are younger gay men. Old, straight businessmen are often uncomfortable with that. When another old straight businessman like me came in, they opened right up. Not once did I get a negative response from the business community. They wanted to shed that image of tough, insensitive businessmen, to show that they understand the problem — but they didn't know how.

Satisfied that I could be productive, I began my one-year leave of absence. I explained my plans to employees, customers, and investors. They were universally supportive.

My first goal was to help produce Aid & Comfort events in other cities. We made a documentary film of the Boston fundraiser, and wrote a manual describing what we did. With those tools, and using my home as an office, I found people in Santa Fe who wanted to develop an Aid & Comfort benefit there. Six more are in the planning stages. I've also spent time coordinating with several local organizations: Strongest Link, an AIDS-care service on Boston's North Shore; and a hot-meals program for PWAs in the Boston area. As I enter the second half of my year-long sabbatical, I'm looking for ways to work with small businesses that can so easily be overwhelmed by the challenges of AIDS.

As for Harbor Sweets? *I* knew my management team could run it perfectly well without me. Now the managers and employees know it too. The business is strong, and it will be stronger still when I return. And no one will doubt that it can continue to thrive once I get hit by a truck.

One of the miracles that is America is the way our country responds to crises. Witness how corporate executives became government leaders in World War II. How we mobilized forces to catch up in our space program and put Americans on the moon. And, more recently, how the nation rallied to reduce the impact of a critical energy crisis.

The AIDS crisis has the potential to cause more devastation than any event in our nation's history. The report of Admiral Watkins and the President's Commission on AIDS recommended specific and logical action, with a compelling sense of wisdom and urgency that is hard to ignore. But most of us have not yet recognized the crisis proportions of this epidemic. AIDS was rarely mentioned in the 1988 presidential campaign, and few of our nation's elected leaders seem personally committed to addressing it. Why are they denying the size of this crisis?

Dr. James Curran of the Centers for Disease Control gives us a clue. He believes the stumbling block is the long incubation period (up to ten years, possibly more) of the AIDS virus. We do not feel the sense of urgency that we do from more immediate tragedies. That is precisely why stronger leadership is so desperately needed. As corporate executives, we have the experience to provide some of that leadership.

Not everyone can take a year away from a job. But if the possibility appeals to you, give it some thought before you decide it's impossible. I did, and the results were so positive, not only for my personal satisfaction and growth but for my business, that I've committed to doing it again in 1994. And if any of you reading this would like to devote your sabbatical to work on AIDS issues, I'd be happy to discuss it with you.

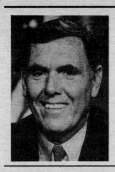

Raymond L. Flynn

WHAT A CARING CITY CAN DO ABOUT AIDS

Raymond L. Flynn is the mayor of Boston and a member of the Task Force on AIDS of the U.S. Conference of Mayors.

THE AIDS EPIDEMIC is now the number one public-health crisis facing this nation. AIDS should be of special concern to elected officials in America's large urban centers. Medical experts estimate that nearly three-quarters of all known AIDS cases in the United States are confined to the nation's twenty most populous cities. Whether the people of our nation will survive the AIDS epidemic, and whether our children will see the eradication of this disease in their lifetime, could very well depend on how wisely and how decisively our cities respond to the challenge that AIDS represents.

First and foremost, elected officials must recognize that AIDS is a medical problem. We must be careful not to let this deadly virus be seen as a political problem or as a civil-rights problem. Urban leaders must enlist the help of the medical experts in their cities to educate urban communities and local officials about AIDS. Officials must develop effective and straightforward AIDS policies that recognize how the disease is spread and that do not discriminate against people with AIDS.

With these policies for guidance, we must develop programs that address all aspects of the issue.

Education: We must send clear and persistent messages on how people can prevent themselves and others from getting infected with the disease. Educational outreach does work, as the gay and lesbian community has demonstrated through their significant efforts. Gay men, once in the highest at-risk behavior group, are no longer the fastest-growing group of HIV-infected individuals. As part of the educational effort in Boston, we have:

• disseminated information on a community-wide basis. For example, we mailed Surgeon General Koop's report on AIDS to every Boston household a full year before the national mailing went out;

• funded community-based agencies that communicate these AIDS messages in a manner that is culturally sensitive and with language that is appropriate to the specific population being addressed. Many of these agencies, such as the AIDS Action Committee, provide both educational outreach and direct services to people with AIDS;

• ensured that our schools adopt a formal curriculum that addresses AIDS issues;

• aggressively reached out to educate those whose behavior places them at high risk of contracting the disease. For example, through our Project Trust program, outreach workers teach IV-drug users about the risks of sharing needles and provide them with bleach to disinfect their needles;

• worked with minority churches throughout the city to coordinate an "AIDS Sunday" during which ministers helped to educate their congregations about the facts of AIDS. Health professionals spoke at churches and AIDS educational literature was distributed throughout Boston's minority community.

Health Care: AIDS is enormously expensive to treat, but we must provide the highest quality care to persons with AIDS in a compassionate and professional fashion. In Boston, we have:

• expanded services at Boston City Hospital to include a walk-in, outpatient AIDS clinic, and to ensure that people with AIDS are provided quality treatment regardless of their resources and insurance status;

• opened the first-in-the-nation pediatric AIDS respite center at Boston City Hospital, which provides infected children with compassionate, 24-hour care in a home-like atmosphere, and provides parents with counseling and support from the clinic's trained staff;

• helped to establish or fund programs at community health centers that provide services for AIDS patients. Last summer, for example, the Fenway Community Health Center opened the nation's first outpatient HIV treatment center to use aerosol pentamidine;

• helped to establish a community-based AIDS hospice that will provide quality care in a supportive environment;

• committed, given the rapid increase of AIDS among IV-drug users, to end the drug-treatment waiting lists in our city. We have begun to expand the capacity of current drug-treatment facilities and, with clergy and community support, have begun to site new facilities throughout the neighborhoods of Boston;

• initiated legislation to establish a pilot needle-exchange program among IV-drug users — the fastest-growing group of people with AIDS — to take infected needles off the streets and out of the hands of those at high risk of getting the disease and of spreading the disease.

Employment: As an essential component of an overall policy that treats everyone with dignity and respect, and serves as a model for other employers, we must ensure that the rules of the municipal workplace protect people with AIDS. In Boston we have:

• promulgated an executive order which prohibits discrimination against city employees with AIDS or those perceived to be in high-risk groups, offering legal protections in cases of harassment or denial of employment benefits;

• conducted training programs for employees at all levels of city government concerning the facts about AIDS and the impact of the executive order which prohibits discrimination.

Clearly the AIDS issue demands immediate and sustained action. Urban leaders must be resourceful and committed in their responses, utilizing multiple strategies to address an increasingly complex issue. Most importantly, they must not let politics get in the way of solving a medical crisis. They must let themselves be guided by the best medical data and not by political expediency.

Perhaps the most important role elected officials in our cities can play in fighting the AIDS epidemic is simply to provide clear and consistent leadership. Those involved in the battle against this most serious epidemic must show by their actions as well as their words their commitment to addressing the problem.

AIDS will not go away if we turn our backs out of ignorance and fear. Elected officials — especially those in areas where the AIDS epidemic is most acute — are morally obligated to lead the way in forging a tolerant and compassionate response to this deadly disease. AIDS challenges not only our physical selves, but the moral fiber of our community as well. It is up to all of us to ensure the survival of both.

Smaller cities, perhaps not yet faced with a dramatic number of people with AIDS, must not sit on their hands until a crisis level of infection is reached. They must begin now to develop comprehensive education and health-care programs so that no one will develop this deadly disease out of ignorance, and so that no one with the disease will face a terminal illness without the compassionate care that he or she deserves.

Bill McBride
RAISING FUNDS FOR AIDS SERVICES

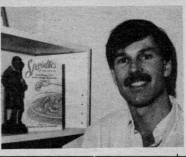

Bill McBride has served as a reading and curriculum specialist in places as diverse as North Carolina and West Germany. He is presently an editor for a major textbook company in Chicago.

I MOVED TO CHICAGO in September 1986. Like many newcomers to a big city, I went looking for fun, for friendship, for the meaning of life, or for some kind of love in crowded bars. As luck would have it, one night a person approached me and asked if I would buy a raffle ticket.

"What for?"

"For Chicago House, a residence for people with AIDS."

"Well, sure, I'll buy one ... But isn't there something else I could do?"

Two weeks later I nervously fumbled with the doorknob of a large old house. I had come to cook my first of many Monday-night meals for people whom I had never seen, for people with AIDS. Over the months, the residents joked that I should write a cookbook. One night I realized how good an idea that was. And one year after that first Monday-night meal we celebrated the publication of *Specialties of the House: Great Recipes from Great Chicago Restaurants*.

In two months we sold over six thousand copies. The profits for Chicago House on the first printing alone should be around $40,000. Such a success comes by following a few essential guidelines.

• *Think about what kind of fundraiser makes sense for you.* For me, it was a cookbook. For someone else, it might be a simple block party, inviting neighbors to drop by for an event and to make a contribution at the same time. A more ambitious group might organize a fundraising walk, where donors pledge a certain amount per mile to people who are walking. These walks have the added benefit that they give participants an easy opening to approach relatives, co-workers, and even strangers on the street about AIDS fundraising.

• *Don't let that good idea die.* When you think you have a good idea, tell someone. Share your idea to build excitement around it, to gather supporters for it, to refine it, to keep it alive. I knew the project was viable after I discussed it with my friend Jim LiSacchi, a native Chicagoan, writer and editor, and gourmet cook. Jim found the idea exciting and wanted to help.

• *Get support and advice from people who know.* How do you begin to put a cookbook together? How do you do anything you've never done before? You find the experts, and you ask them for advice. We contacted the food editors of the Chicago *Sun Times*, the Chicago *Tribune*, and *Chicago Magazine*, and the managers of three prominent restaurants. All gave us good adviceand , names of people to contact for help, and most importantly, all agreed to let us use their names and those of their institutions on any promotional material we produced.

• *Don't stop because you don't know all the answers.* The more we found out, the more we found out we didn't know. How would we get hundreds of recipes home tested? How would we find an inexpensive but good printer, paper company, sales company, and distributor? What about marketing, financing, and copyright laws?

You should not be embarrassed by your ignorance. Just keep asking and take notes. By July we had a printer who would do the job at thirty percent below cost, a paper company that would give us the paper at cost, a distributor that donated all the profits on mail order, a sales company whose salespeople donated their six-percent commission, and a lawyer who reviewed our contracts and registered our copyright for free.

•*Network within and outside of your community.* Don't limit your contacts. And don't sell people short. Compassion is a universal human quality. We were repeatedly surprised at people's openness and willingness to offer their time, money, expertise, and resources to help people with AIDS. If you run into the occasional negative person, don't let it stop you. Keep your sense of humor, and keep telling everyone about your project.

An artist I met over a milkshake at Goodies toy store suggested that I call his boss. After one meeting, McKnight Design offered to do the illustrations, cover art, and keylining, as well as get us a typesetter — at no cost. Jim LiSacchi met Jeff Smith, the *Frugal Gourmet*, at an Art Institute party for restaurant owners. After a simple explanation, Jeff enthusiastically agreed to write the foreword to the book.

Three cooking schools and sixty of my fellow employees offered to test nearly two hundred recipes. Mary Schafer, a co-worker and production coordinator, agreed to design the book and to oversee the production. Editors Ron Rutkowski and Teri Firmiss volunteered months of their time to put the book together.

•*Call people back. Go see them again. Then follow up some more.* Be pleasantly persistent. We had estimated that by June 15 we would have over 150 recipes. We had 23. For the next two months we walked the streets and called people every day. By August, in order to meet deadlines, we stopped; at that point we had 91 restaurants and 160 recipes.

•*Market your product or project.* You must be a salesperson. Call radio and television stations once you have something exciting and tangible to show them. Make contacts with newspaper and magazine people. Never stop selling your idea. Speaking of selling, you can order a cookbook (ask for *Specialties of the House*) for $9.95 plus $2.00 postage and handling by calling Independent Publishers Group at 1-800-888-4741!

•*Say "Thank You!"* You can't thank people enough. Call

people back. Write them thank-you notes. If there is a question about listing someone in a credit, list them. People need to be acknowledged and told that their compassion is appreciated.

One person I would like to thank is a certain volunteer who approached me a year ago wanting money for something called Chicago House. I never did find much fun that night. But I did learn something about the meaning of life. By giving and helping others, you can find a lifetime of love and friendship. Not bad for one raffle ticket.

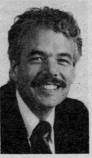
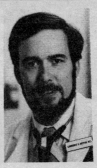

Lawrence Deyton
& John Y. Killen, Jr.
VOLUN-
TEERING
FOR A
STUDY

Dr. Lawrence Deyton, better known as "Bopper," and Dr. John Y. Killen, Jr., are both involved in AIDS research at the National Institute of Allergy and Infectious Diseases (NIAID).

OVER THE PAST FEW YEARS, a tremendous amount of time and money has gone into medical research aimed at halting the spread of AIDS. Much of this research is aimed at one of two goals:

(1) Treatments for people already infected with the AIDS virus. The most urgent need, of course, is treatment for those individuals who are already ill. In addition, we're investigating what drugs, if any, may prevent someone already infected with the HIV virus from coming down with AIDS. Often, the same drugs are being studied for both purposes.

(2) Vaccines for people not currently infected. We must find a vaccine that will protect people from becoming infected with the AIDS virus. If and when such a vaccine is found, it could quickly provide protection for much of the world's population, and might ultimately allow us to eradicate AIDS entirely, just as we have wiped out the once-feared smallpox virus.

The early development and testing of these treatments can be done without human subjects. But eventually, every promising drug or treatment must be tested in the population for whom it is intended. There is no other way to be sure of its effectiveness and side effects. Until a vaccine and a cure are found, we will need volunteers for these clinical trials.

Drug tests: These trials involve volunteers who have tested positive for HIV antibodies. There are trials which focus on people who have ARC (AIDS-Related Complex) or full-blown AIDS as well as people who have no symptoms of their HIV infection. Naturally, anyone who has HIV infection is going to want the best possible treatment for themselves. At this point, we are beginning to have a clear idea of exactly what that is. Much more work needs to be done. A drug that looks good at first may turn out to have highly toxic long-term effects. One that doesn't show much short-term effect may ultimately be very beneficial. The main requirement for volunteers in HIV drug tests is a commitment to stay with it even if the results aren't immediately promising. Understandably, many people with HIV infection will not feel comfortable making such a commitment. But for those who do, there are benefits: not only the opportunity to help in the race to find a cure for AIDS, but the possibility that they will be among the first people to be helped by a new medication that proves effective. In addition, all volunteers benefit from high-quality care in a field that is rapidly changing. Clinical research on AIDS is supported by the federal government, private industry, and by philanthropic organizations and takes place both at large medical centers and in community settings such as doctors' offices, hospitals, and clinics.

Vaccine tests: The purpose of a vaccine, unlike a cure, is to prevent a person from becoming infected with a virus. Volunteers for AIDS vaccine tests should have a normal immune system and must not already be infected. That is, they should test negative for the AIDS antibody. Anyone meeting those criteria is a possible candidate for such trials. One complication of vaccine tests is that they will usually cause a person to register positive for the AIDS antibodies on the most commonly available tests. All such volunteers are supplied with certificates explaining their situation, and more elaborate antibody tests will reveal that they are not actually infected with the AIDS virus. However, they risk some possibility of discrimination because of their HIV-positive status.

Clearly, no one should volunteer for either type of study without thoroughly understanding both the possible risks and the possible benefits of such an action. The researchers responsible for the study should provide such counseling to potential volunteers. Additional information can be obtained from the private or government sponsor of the trial.

FOLLOW-UP:

Anyone interested in the possibility of participating in such tests should check with their local AIDS organization or city or county health department to see if there are studies in the area that need volunteers. The AIDS Clinical Trials Information Service, at 1-800-TRIALS-A, provides current information on federally and privately sponsored clinical trials for AIDS patients and others infected with HIV. This free service is a Public Health Service project provided collaboratively by the Centers for Disease Control, the Food and Drug Administration, the National Institute of Allergy and Infectious Diseases, and the National Library of Medicine. The American Foundation for AIDS Research (see appendix) also publishes a directory of drug trials being conducted by government, academic, industry, and community-based organizations.

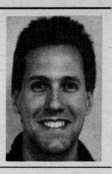

Tom Soles
STARTING AN AIDS HOTLINE

Tom Soles is coordinator of the Minnesota AIDS Line, a volunteer-based counseling, information, and referral line. He has supervised volunteer counselors on a separate general crisis hotline, and has provided education for teenagers about sexuality and communication.

THE ISSUES THAT SURROUND the AIDS crisis are the very issues that many of us have learned not to talk about: sexuality, drug use, disease, and death. Because of this, anonymous, non-judgmental, reliable AIDS hotlines have become a vital part of the fight against AIDS; phone counseling is very accessible and also very "safe," meaning that a caller doesn't have to worry about what the person at the other end of the phone line thinks about his or her questions.

The first step in starting a hotline, though, is to decide whether a new phone service is needed. Does your city or region already have a hotline that is providing AIDS-related counseling, information, and referral? Even if the answer is no, it may be that adding AIDS-information resources to an existing phone service makes more sense than starting a separate service.

You will want to meet with representatives from nearby social-service organizations to determine how best to respond to the needs in your area. This cooperation will allow you to maximize organizing, recruiting, and publicity efforts.

Once you've decided that a new telephone service is needed, or that an existing service should be expanded, think about the scope of your service. Will it provide information? Referrals? Counseling? Whatever the stated purpose of your line, however — even if it is merely the office phone for a local AIDS task force — you *will* receive phone calls for all these things. Anticipating those phone calls will make your job easier.

Thorough planning is the next step. Hundreds of other AIDS hotlines have already been set up around the country, so don't try to plan "from scratch." Talk with others about their experiences. The National AIDS Network (see appendix) publishes a directory of AIDS hotlines which will make research much easier. In addition, networking with non-AIDS-related hotlines in your area can give you some valuable information.

Drawing on the work of Rick Grossman, who has started hotlines in Philadelphia and Houston, I'll briefly touch on some aspects that will need to be a part of planning your phone line:

• *Careful screening and training of the telephone staff.* Not all people who volunteer will actually be effective counselors; there are many ways to fight AIDS, and the energies of some will be better used in other areas. Counselors must have the ability to remain non-judgmental toward callers. We all have values and beliefs, but not imposing them on clients is a vital part of helping. The only "directives" given by counselors should be advocating risk reduction. Other qualities to look for are listening skills, openness, honesty, empathy, and an ability to separate their own experiences and pain from those of the caller. In addition to working on those skills, training will need to include values exploration, crisis-intervention methods, ethics, confidentiality, information on local resources, and a chance to practice phone work with role-plays.

• *Referrals.* Beyond providing AIDS information and counseling, referrals will be the next most important aspect of a hotline. Other AIDS organizations, state and local health departments, the local Red Cross, testing sites, and crisis-intervention centers can help you develop your referral listings.

• *Use and Supervision of Volunteers.* Using trained volunteers will have a number of benefits. Their donated time will allow you to have two or more lines, keeping your phone service accessible to callers. Many people want to give their time and energy to the AIDS crisis; involving these people as volunteer counselors is rewarding both for you and your community. Counselors need and deserve support in what they do; it can be a tough job. If a supervisor isn't always present, one should be on call. Volunteers should have a way to check in with someone after a shift is worked.

• *Documentation of Calls.* You'll need a way to track who you are serving, to measure growth and changes, and to show the need for your service and back-up funding efforts. This probably means asking volunteers to fill out a form after each call; these forms can then be tallied at the end of each month.

• *Public Relations.* You might want to your publicity before your line actually starts service so that volunteers are getting calls from the start. While posters, brochures, photocopied flyers, and cards will be important P.R. tools, a good relationship with your local media will be of primary importance. This could start with simply contacting newspapers, radio, and TV stations, letting them know that you are a resource that they can give their audiences in connection with articles or features about AIDS. You might want to consider a press conference with press kits outlining your new hotline. There are many good books on the subject, one of which is *The Publicity Handbook* by David R. Yale.

• *Fundraising.* The best bet here is finding someone who has experience in grant writing and fundraising. Some beginning resources, though, might be community health organizations to look for donated office space, and communications companies that might donate your phones and the cost of setting them up.

Clearly this is a beginning outline, something to get you

thinking about the possibilities. It can be done, and there is a great deal of support and guidance available through already existing hotlines and agencies. The need for hotlines as central sources of caring, sensitivity, and reliable information will continue to be a critical part of America's response to AIDS.

RESOURCES:

For more suggestions about starting an AIDS hotline, call the Minnesota AIDS Line at 612-870-0700.

TAKING ACTION IN MINORITY COMMUNITIES

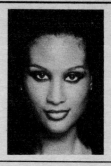

Beverly Johnson is an actress and one of the world's foremost fashion models; in 1974 she became the first black woman to appear on the cover of Vogue *magazine. She appears with Ron Reagan and Ruben Blades in the film* AIDS: Changing the Rules.

IN PREPARING THIS CHAPTER, I interviewed one of the most inspiring women I have ever met: Dr. Rita Webb Smith. Miss Rita, as she is affectionately called, has also been called the urban Harriet Tubman and a living miracle worker. She organized her neighbors — mostly women and children — to form the 143rd Street Preservation Group in New York City. Together they declared war on the drug dealers and users who had taken over their neighborhood. "Now," Miss Rita says, "we have to deal with AIDS."

Miss Rita, along with three people from the community and myself, have begun outlining the steps that need to be taken in the Harlem community and in every community throughout the United States that suffers from rampant drug abuse — communities which therefore also suffer from the sharing of infected needles, which is the surest way to contract AIDS.

The most important thing needed in minority communities around the nation is information. We blacks and Hispanics remain woefully uninformed about ways to prevent a disease that is, or soon will be, killing hundreds of thousands of us, gay and straight, male and female, young and old. Fortunately, there are things we can do:

• *Inform yourself.* Be sure you know what you're talking about. Contact a local AIDS-related group in or near where you live and ask for information. Read the newspapers. Giving out wrong information may be worse than doing nothing.

• *Support community-based organizations.* No one likes a person from somewhere else telling him or her how to act — the most effective way to help a community is from inside the community. Most major cities have at least one community-based organization devoted to the AIDS-related needs of minorities. Find it. The need for volunteers in minority communities is even more acute than elsewhere. If you have skills or resources that might help spread the word about AIDS, be sure to let the organization know. This can be anything from an ability to write a clear newsletter to using your connections with local media — black or Spanish radio stations or newspapers. Maybe you know how to put an ad campaign together. Maybe your sister or co-worker does.

• *Make use of block associations.* A block-by-block movement can help get people organized. Parent associations are important organizations to address the AIDS problem. Start a local health fair with the main focus on AIDS. Perhaps you can get funding or support for mobile units where people can seek information on AIDS, and also be tested for AIDS.

• *If there isn't a community-based organization, start one up.* This won't be easy, but it's important. You'll need lots of savvy with city political machinery, red tape, and grant forms. Look for unoccupied city or state office space. Find local leaders — religious leaders (the church is an important influence in black communities), popular politicians, neighborhood businessmen — and get their support. Ask shops to donate their services, or window space for signs. Talk to similar organizations in other cities to see what they do. Make sure the local hotline number is visible all over town.

• *Speak out for causes that will help.* Learn as much as you can about campaigns to distribute information, clean needles, bleach (for disinfecting needles), or free condoms to addicts; or movements to include clear, unequivocating AIDS education in public schools; or ways to improve the quality of care in our inner-city hospitals. Do your best to sort out the pros and cons of these causes. Again, talk to local AIDS-related groups — ask questions and hear what they have to say. Then, get active. Many chapters in this book can help you.

These are some of the principles that Dr. Rita Webb Smith has used in organizing the highly successful 143rd Street Preservation Group. The same principles can be valuable for any group in fighting the AIDS epidemic.

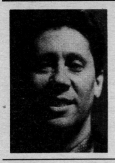

Mitchell Cutler
STARTING A BUDDY PROGRAM

Mitchell Cutler is the founder of the Gay Men's Health Crisis Buddy Program, the first program of its kind. He is a native New Yorker and a rare-book dealer.

IN 1982, I STARTED THE Gay Men's Health Crisis Buddy Program. The idea was to connect individual volunteers — buddies — with PWAs (people with AIDS) who might benefit from the friendship and support that a buddy could provide.

These buddies, it was felt, could provide a myriad of services for PWAs and their families: running errands, making hospital visits, walking dogs, translating for parents and doctors, cleaning homes, and offering general support by using common sense and compassion to enable PWAs to proceed with their lives in a dignified and more independent manner.

In the years that the buddy program has been in operation, we've learned a great deal. Here are a few thoughts for anyone else trying to establish a similar program:

• Communication is the key to successfully establishing a buddy program in a new region. Use every opportunity to solicit volunteers: Put up signs on bulletin boards in supermarkets, medical centers, community centers, health clubs, universities, health-food stores, and meeting places for gay groups; contact all the local media; speak before civic, religious, and social clubs; inform the local hotline services about your existence. Volunteers can be old, young, male, female, English-

and non-English-speaking, professionals, retirees, house-wives, college students, gay, and straight.

• A training and selection process is a vital part of any program. An excellent model is explained in the National AIDS Network's volunteer training manual. A good training program will need to cover many areas, ranging from health and safety guidelines to role-playing in preparation for the situations buddies will encounter.

• A buddy program will not be successful until people with AIDS are involved in its planning and operation.

• The program will require a coordinator. The coordinator, or someone well informed about the program and able to reach the coordinator, should be available, on-call, 24 hours a day. Emergencies don't happen on a nine-to-five schedule.

• Both the coordinator and the volunteers must accept their limitations. Not all requests for help can be filled.

• Get in touch, and stay in touch, with other agencies that may already be serving PWAs: hospitals, churches, drug-rehabilitation centers, and social-service groups. Figure out how you can work with them to provide the best buddy system.

• The program we set up in New York was the first of its kind, and we had to learn a great deal by trial and error. You don't need to go through that. Get in touch with the nearest existing buddy system and see how you can learn from their experiences. Perhaps members of your group can go through their training session, or a representative from their program can come to your planning meetings, or they can provide you with copies of the materials they use at their training sessions. None of us is alone in doing this. Only by sharing our resources and knowledge can we accomplish all that needs to be done.

FOLLOW-UP:

The "Volunteer Management" manual mentioned above is available from the National AIDS Network, 2033 M St. NW, Suite 800, Washington, DC 20036; 202-293-2437. The cost is $5.00 for NAN members and $15.00 for non-members.

Michael Callen
C.R.I.s:
A CREATIVE
APPROACH TO
AIDS RESEARCH

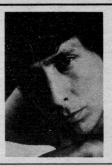

Michael Callen was diagnosed seven years ago with AIDS. He is a founding member of the People with AIDS Coalition (New York), and the Community Research Initiative. In his non-AIDS life, he is a singer and songwriter whose album Purple Heart *was recently released.*

EIGHT YEARS into the AIDS epidemic, only one drug for the treatment of AIDS, AZT, has made it through the maze of federal research regulations — and I believe AZT will ultimately prove to be a far more dangerous drug than most people now believe. Why is this the best that federal treatment research has been able to produce?

In November 1986, something extraordinary happened. For the first time in history, a group of people *with* a disease organized to sponsor treatment research to help save their own lives. Rather than continue butting our heads up against a wall of federal indifference and incompetence, we decided to stop trying to figure out how to solve the federal treatment logjam. Instead, people with AIDS and ARC decided to roll up our sleeves and take matters into our own hands. In mid-1987, the People with AIDS Coalition in New York formed the Community Research Initiative and began enrolling subjects in treatment trials. Similar attempts to organize research initiatives based in the affected communities have sprung up in San Francisco and Atlanta. People in other cities with large AIDS populations are now exploring the possibility of starting their own treatment research initiatives.

Starting your own community research initiative is a less daunting task than it may seem at first. All that is required is sufficient political will plus enough money to hire an administrator, rent some office space, and hook up some telephones. In the United States, most drug research is done by the government or in large medical centers. But the AIDS crisis was so great that we looked at this system and found a major resource that was not being tapped: the expertise and practices of community physicians with large AIDS and ARC practices. Because these physicians are responsible for the day-to-day management of patient care, they have insights and expertise which have not been utilized by those in the federal agencies who are designing AIDS treatment trials from their academic ivory towers. Community physicians also have the trust of their patients, which means that the data they collect is likely to be more reliable.

How can you support the idea of community research initiatives? First, find out if there is already one formed or forming in your area. If there is, call and ask what you can do to help. Send a donation; volunteer time.

If there isn't a Community Research Initiative in your area, why not form a committee to explore the feasibility of forming one? The Community Research Initiative of New York has a "starter pack" of materials for people interested in organizing their own CRIs.

Briefly, a Community Research Initiative needs four components:

1. *An administrative component*, to coordinate efforts. An administrative director does fundraising, and community relations, handles correspondence between the other components of CRI, and generally is responsible for all the detail work and record keeping.

2. *An Institutional Review Board (IRB)*, to comply with federal regulations. An IRB is made up of representatives from

the community (lawyers, clergy, women, men, people of color, people with AIDS, etc.) who review research proposals with a concern for protecting the subjects who may participate in that protocol. The IRB asks these questions: Is the risk taken by the research subject justified by the potential benefit to the patient and society at large? Is there any way to reduce these risks without compromising the potential research benefits? Is the informed consent form clear and easily understood? Will confidentiality be adequately protected? In its simplest terms, the IRB puts itself in the shoes of a potential research subject and asks: Would *I* feel safe being involved in this study? An IRB can demand changes in the protocol and in the language of the informed consent. In the United States, no research on human subjects can take place until an IRB has reviewed and approved the protocol as ethical. For this reason, the IRB is very important and very powerful.

3. *An Executive Scientific Committee*, made up of community physicians and respected AIDS researchers from your local area. They review for scientific merit protocols submitted to the CRI; they can also generate their own protocols. Like the IRB, they are powerful because they can either reject a protocol, approve a protocol, or recommend specific changes. Because CRIs are currently such an exciting concept, you should have no trouble attracting top-notch scientific expertise to this committee.

4. *Community physicians* who are willing to participate and to recommend to their own patients that they become involved in CRI trials. These physicians are the most important part of your CRI Program.

The best way to form a CRI within your own community is to begin publicizing your intent. Place an ad in local newspapers seeking others interested in forming a CRI. Call up the major AIDS service-providing organizations and tell them you're interested in forming a committee to explore the idea of forming a CRI. Or ask a few people with AIDS to identify some of the major AIDS researchers and doctors. Then be bold: Call them up and invite them to join your committee.

Identify a lawyer who is familiar with FDA regulations and state regulations. Ask the lawyer (who may be willing to work for free) to write an opinion letter on what city, state, and federal regulations might govern the formation of a CRI in your community.

And then there's that horrible task of fundraising. But money will be needed to hire an administrator and pay for office space and clerical help. Hiring the right administrator is probably the most important choice you'll make. This person must be knowledgeable about AIDS and the drug treatment situation, be good at organizing and fundraising, and have good community-relations skills.

One thing that's special about New York's CRI is that it is a project of the People with AIDS Coalition. This has insured that the people most directly affected by treatment research are involved in its planning and oversight from the beginning. Affiliating with a local PWA organization or having significant input from people with AIDS and ARC will contribute significantly to the success of your CRI.

Americans are an inventive people. Our country's history has proven time and again that when we *really* want to get something accomplished, we find a way to do it. Let the federal research efforts continue along at their sluggish pace. Meanwhile, let's explore our own unique and creative solutions.

FOLLOW-UP:

Community-based clinical trial groups now exist in most major U.S. cities. For a listing of the community-based clinical trial group in your area, phone Paul Corser at the American Foundation for AIDS Research, 212-719-0033.

For further information about how to form your own CRI (or to make a tax-deductible donation to an existing CRI), write: Community Research Initiative, c/o People with AIDS Coalition, 263A West 19th Street, Room 125, New York, NY 10011; 212-532-0290.

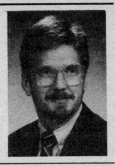

James L. Holm
TAKING THE NEXT STEP

James L. Holm is acting executive director of the National AIDS Network in Washington, D.C.

AS THE AIDS CRISIS PROLIFERATES, more and more people outside this country's major metropolitan areas will be affected. Official projections show AIDS moving into the suburbs and the country. Small towns and rural areas that didn't have to deal with AIDS in the epidemic's early days will be challenged to address the needs of friends, neighbors, relatives, and others whom everyone once assumed to be safely out of reach of the "big-city" plague. Those of a prophetic bent predict that AIDS, and how we respond to it, will define the latter decades of this century in tomorrow's history books.

History will show us to be either the great nation we have been in the past, a nation of individuals who tolerate one another's diversity and demonstrate compassion for their fellow citizens' misfortune — or a nation riven by fear and ignorance. The virus behind the AIDS epidemic has accomplished its insidious purpose by not only directly threatening the lives of well over one hundred thousand Americans, but by tearing at the very fabric of our society as well. AIDS is called the most political of all diseases. Indeed, it pits moralists and ideologues against those who support compassionate, nonjudgmental treatment for those it has afflicted, providing those who seek it a hook on which to hang their personal prejudices.

It pits family members against one another and turns neighbors into adversaries. More than anything before it, AIDS proves that ignorance leads to fear, and knowledge leads to compassion.

Since the beginning of the AIDS crisis, community organizations have taken the lead in battling the disease. Drawing on one of America's finest traditions — communities taking care of their own by contributing money and volunteering time — community-based organizations offer a variety of services to people with AIDS that can include "buddies" to help with household chores and errands, housing for the indigent and those who have been turned out of their own homes, support groups for the infected and those at risk of infection, and assistance with legal matters such as writing wills and procuring Social Security benefits.

More than 650 community-based organizations around the country are involved in providing AIDS-related services. Some were formed specifically to respond to AIDS; others realized that working with AIDS is an appropriate extension of the work they already do. They all share a simple philosophy: that care is best provided at the community level, that diversity must be respected and accommodated, and that the goal of all AIDS services is to uphold the quality of an individual's life by nurturing hope, independence, and self-determination.

It sounds simple and noble enough. But there's a catch. While the number of AIDS cases in the United States increases, the organizations responding to the crisis are taxed beyond all reasonable limits. Funding has been hard to come by. Volunteers have felt overwhelmed. Because AIDS has struck mainly the big cities, those outside the cities — even many within the cities who could delude themselves into feeling immune — have distanced themselves from the disease. Despite assurance from the most credible scientists and health officials this country has that AIDS is not casually transmitted, many Americans still shudder at the thought of seeing, let alone touching or hugging, a person with AIDS.

But living in a cocoon won't be so easy in the years ahead. As the number of Americans now infected with the AIDS virus become tomorrow's people with AIDS, it will be harder to hide from the reality that AIDS is all our problem. It's a problem for our inner cities. It's a problem for hospitals in the hometowns to which many city dwellers return to spend their last days. It will be a more pressing problem in the years ahead for those small towns as residents confront AIDS right next door, down the street — or in their own household.

As you have read throughout this book, AIDS is affecting every part of American life. No one is exempt. No one is immune. Eventually it will affect all of us in one way or another. Given projections that one to two million Americans are now infected with the AIDS virus, it's only a matter of time before someone in our lives, perhaps someone we love very much, will face the challenges of living with AIDS.

We will defeat AIDS and erase its blot on our society only by being informed on how the virus is and is not transmitted, educating others in our community with factual information they can understand and relate to, and stopping the sexual and drug-using practices that put us and others at risk of infection. By getting involved, we can show our concern for individuals affected by AIDS, and uphold the traditions of caring and civic responsibility that have made America the great nation it is. Contributing money to an organization in your community is one way. Volunteering time and professional services is another way.

While there are hundreds of agencies nationwide that offer AIDS-related services, possibly there isn't one in your area. A number of organizations provide visiting-nurse services, "meals on wheels," hospices — traditional agencies that have, in some areas, branched out to include providing services to people with AIDS and other AIDS services. Sufficient community support could generate interest in providing such services so they will be in place when they become necessary. The first step is finding out what is already offered locally. Talk to those agencies. Talk to community, business, and religious leaders. Organize a group of local activists who can stir up interest.

Call us. The National AIDS Network represents the 650-plus community-based organizations around the United States involved in providing AIDS-related services. As the national clearinghouse and resource center for these organizations, we can put you in touch with your local health clinic, social-service agency, church group, or other organization, which will be happy to hear from you and to discuss how you can assist them and become one of the troops who have declared war on AIDS.

However you decide to help, you will be rewarded with the satisfaction of knowing you are part of a nationwide network of people who care. If you don't yet know of an organization in your community that provides services to people with AIDS, or other AIDS services to the community at large, please contact us.

FOLLOW-UP:

The National AIDS Network is at 2033 M St. NW, Suite 800, Washington, DC 20036; 202-293-AIDS.

APPENDIX

DIRECTORY OF
AIDS-RELATED
ORGANIZATIONS

Compiled by Steven Zorn

AIDS ACTION COUNCIL, 2033 M St. NW, Suite 801, Washington, DC 20036; 202-293-2886.

This national organization works with the federal government to create a sound national AIDS policy and lobbies for funding for AIDS research and treatment. It represents more than 700 community-based organizations that provide direct services to people with AIDS.

AIDS COALITION TO UNLEASH POWER (ACT UP), 496A Hudson St., Suite G4, New York, NY 10014; 212-989-1114. (Consult your phone book for your local chapter.)

ACT UP is a diverse, non-partisan group committed to direct action to end the AIDS crisis. ACT UP meets with government and public officials, researches and distributes the latest medical information, and organizes protests and demonstrations. ACT UP/New York provides small grants and sends speakers and information to emerging AIDS-activist organizations. There are ACT UP chapters in more than fifty cities.

AMERICAN ASSOCIATION OF PHYSICIANS FOR HUMAN RIGHTS (AAPHR), 2940 16th St., #105, San Francisco, CA 94103; 415-255-4547.

AAPHR is a national organization of physicians and medical students that deals with medical issues affecting homosexual men and women. While not specifically an AIDS organization, AAPHR releases position statements about various AIDS issues such as national mandatory antibody testing, airline discrimination against people with AIDS, and AIDS as a women's and minority issue. It also runs a national referral service used by physicians and patients.

AMERICAN FOUNDATION FOR AIDS RESEARCH (AmFAR), 5900 Wilshire Blvd., 2nd Floor, East Satellite, Los Angeles, CA 90036; 213-857-5900; and 1515 Broadway, Suite 3601, New York, NY 10036; 212-719-0033.

AmFAR is the nation's leading private-sector funding organization dedicated to AIDS research, education, and public policy. Eighty percent of AmFAR's grants underwrite scientific research to find a vaccine and effective treatments for AIDS. Twenty percent of the grants go toward experimental educational programs to prevent the spread of the disease. AmFAR publishes an AIDS/HIV experimental treatment directory, which is available free to PWAs, PWARCs, their advocates, and AIDS professionals. It also publishes a business guide to AIDS education.

THE AMERICAN RED CROSS, 17th and D Streets, Washington, DC 20006; 202-639-3223. (Consult your phone book for your local chapter.)

The objective of the American Red Cross is to slow the spread of AIDS through information and education that encourages responsible behavior. It provides training and educational materials for use in schools, in the workplace, and for minorities and the general public, as well as other forms of support to people with AIDS, their families, and people testing HIV-positive. Contact your local chapter, as listed in the phone book, for these materials.

COMPUTERIZED AIDS INFORMATION NETWORK (CAIN), Gay and Lesbian Community Service Center, 1213 North Highland Ave., Los Angeles, CA 90038; 213-854-3006.

This computer database provides AIDS information to

subscribers twenty-four hours a day. The Network receives five thousand articles each month; the information is constantly updated. Listings in CAIN are free. The Network also allows people to communicate with one another anonymously via computer. It is funded by the State of California.

MOTHERS OF AIDS PATIENTS (MAP), P.O. Box 3132, San Diego, CA 92103; 619-544-0430.

MAP was started by three mothers who have lost children to AIDS. It offers emotional support to families of people with AIDS, provides information about the disease, and assists people with AIDS who have been rejected by or are isolated from their families. It gives referrals and support by phone or mail. Funding is through private donations.

THE NAMES PROJECT, P.O. Box 14573, 2362 Market St., San Francisco, CA 94114; 415-863-5511.

The Names Project sponsors the AIDS Memorial Quilt. The Quilt serves to illustrate the humanity behind the statistics, provides comfort and a positive expression of grief to those who have been directly affected by the epidemic, and raises money for service agencies that provide care to PWAs and their families. There are local chapters of The Names Project and 8,500 volunteers nationwide. Funding is through private donations.

NATIONAL AIDS NETWORK, 2033 M St. NW, Suite 800, Washington, DC 20036; 202-293-2437.

The National AIDS Network consists of community-based AIDS organizations, hospitals, and educational facilities. It provides technical assistance, grants, and referral services to its member organizations. It is funded through private donations.

NATIONAL ASSOCIATION OF PEOPLE WITH AIDS, 2025 I Street NW, Suite 1118, Washington, DC 20005; 202-429-2856.

NAPWA is an association of local organizations by and for people with AIDS. It is based on the philosophy of self-empowerment. The Association provides information and referrals to its member organizations and also advocates for rights for people with AIDS. It has more than 102 affiliates. Funding is through private donations and foundations.

NATIONAL COUNCIL OF CHURCHES/AIDS TASK FORCE, 475 Riverside Dr., Room 572, New York, NY 10115; 212-870-2421.

Preventive education is the focus of this group; it has compiled a resource and information packet for use by religious leaders in their congregations.

NATIONAL LEADERSHIP COALITION ON AIDS, 1150 17th St. NW, Suite 202, Washington, DC 20036; 202-429-0930.

The National Leadership Coalition on AIDS was formed in May 1987 to consolidate corporate, labor, and civic support in response to the HIV epidemic. The Coalition represents over 170 corporations, labor groups, and prominent voluntary sector organizations responding to AIDS. The Coalition has recently received a five-year grant from the Centers for Disease Control to increase AIDS awareness and prevention among minority and small businesses.

FURTHER READING:
THE BEST BOOKS
ABOUT AIDS

Selected by the editor

SCIENTIFIC AND MEDICAL KNOWLEDGE of AIDS and treatments for AIDS is still changing rapidly. Books are not the best source of up-to-date medical information, but on other aspects of AIDS they can provide a depth of information that is impossible to find elsewhere. For this bibliography we selected books that are tops in their field, and a few others of special significance.

Only AIDS-related books are listed here. For follow-up in other areas such as fundraising, a well-stocked bookstore or library should be helpful.

AIDS: A self-care manual, by AIDS Project Los Angeles, edited by BettyClare Moffatt, Judith Spiegel, Steve Parrish, and Michael Helquiest. IBS Press, 1987. Paperback, 306 pages, $12.95.

Put out by one of the country's leading AIDS service organizations, this comprehensive guide for people with AIDS covers nutrition, finances and benefits (including insurance, disability coverage, and Social Security), and spiritual concerns. This book is often recommended by AIDS organizations for their clients, and will be useful to both PWAs and those who care for them.

AIDS AND ITS METAPHORS, by Susan Sontag. Farrar Straus Giroux, 1988. Cloth, 95 pages, $14.95.

In this long essay, Sontag contends that the words and

metaphors we use to describe AIDS have prevented us from responding to it as we should. Her conclusions put a useful perspective on the question of why there is often too much paranoia, and too little practical action.

AIDS AND THE LAW: A guide for the public, edited by Harlon Dalton, Scott Burris, and the Yale AIDS Law Project. Yale University Press, 1987. Paperback, 382 pages, unpriced.

This comprehensive guide will be mainly of interest to legal professionals, though it is also accessible to interested non-lawyers. The contributors explore the way the legal system currently responds to AIDS issues, and make recommendations on what should be done, in areas such as insurance, screening workers for AIDS, schoolchildren with AIDS, prostitution, and the right to medical treatment.

THE AIDS CAREGIVER'S HANDBOOK, ed. by Ted Eidson. St. Martin's, 1988. Paperback, 330 pages, $10.95.

Eidson has compiled materials developed by the AIDS Project of the Oak Lawn Counseling Center in Dallas, to create a useful manual for anyone who provides care for someone with AIDS or ARC, whether in a professional or personal context. Advice ranges from the practical — how do you change sheets without disturbing the person in bed? — to psychological and interpersonal concerns.

AIDS: Personal stories in pastoral perspective, by Earl Shelp, Ronald H. Sunderland, and Peter W.A. Mansell. The Pilgrim Press, 1986. Paperback, 205 pages, $7.95.

The authors charge that the near-total failure of the church to fill its mandated role in responding to AIDS raises questions about the integrity of contemporary American Christendom. By focusing on the actual experiences of people with AIDS, they show what role the church has played — or failed to play. From this, they suggest ways that the religious community can better meet the challenge of AIDS.

AIDS: The women, ed. by Ines Rieder and Patricia Ruppelt. Cleis, 1988. Paperback, 252 pages, $9.95.

By examining the many ways that AIDS has affected them as women, the women represented here put a personal face on the AIDS tragedy. The diverse contributors include health workers, prostitutes, mothers and sisters of people with AIDS, and IV-drug users.

AIDS: Trading fears for facts; a guide for teens, by Karen Hein, M.D. and Theresa Foy DiGeronimo. Consumer Reports Books, 1989. Paperback, 196 pages, $3.95.

The authors provide a solid, factual introduction to the issues that will concern most teenagers, including safer sex, drug use, and the AIDS antibody test. The heavy use of photographs and illustrations should increase the book's appeal for its intended audience. Gay teenagers, however, will find their concerns better covered in other books such as *Lynda Madaras Talks to Teens About AIDS*.

BORROWED TIME: An AIDS memoir, by Paul Monette. Harcourt Brace Jovanovich, 1988. Cloth, 342 pages, $18.95.

Watching a loved one suffer from AIDS is as foreign as being on the moon, writes Paul Monette. His account of the twenty months from his lover's diagnosis to death conveys that experience with unmatched eloquence.

CONFRONTING AIDS: Directions for public health, health care and research, by the Institute of Medicine, National Academy of Science. National Academy Press, 1986. Paperback, 374 pages, $24.95; and **CONFRONTING AIDS: UPDATE 1988,** same author and publisher, 1988. Paperback, 239 pages, $24.95.

These two reports (the update complements, but does not replace, the original one) offer a thorough basis of facts and recommendations for public policy on AIDS. They call for a massive public-health campaign, discuss the medical and economic aspects of the epidemic, and outline several areas of critical research. Because of the prestigiousness of the originating body, these reports will be especially useful for policy-makers in government, health care, and education.

DOES AIDS HURT? Educating young children about AIDS, by Marcia Quackenbush and Sylvia Villarreal. Network Publications, 1988. Paperback, 149 pages, $14.95.

Aimed at parents, teachers, and other adults who work with children (up to age ten), this book suggests ways to raise the subject of AIDS with children, and offers possible answers to the most often asked questions on the subject. The authors emphasize that different responses are appropriate for different age groups, and that for young children, general information about health and hygiene is more important than explicit information about AIDS. They also include a lengthy section of background information for the adult reader.

HOW TO PERSUADE YOUR LOVER TO USE A CONDOM ... AND WHY YOU SHOULD, by Patti Breitman, Kim Knutson, and Paul Reed. Prima Publishing, 1987. Paperback, 84 pages, $4.95.

Because of AIDS, condoms are now being advertised on network television for the first time ever, and have been the subject of several books. The books have all tended toward the superficial (what did you expect from a book focusing entirely on condoms?), but this is as good as any of them. The authors suggest replies to the most common objections to condom use, and provide basic facts about condoms, AIDS, and other sexually-transmitted diseases.

LYNDA MADARAS TALKS TO TEENS ABOUT AIDS, by Lynda Madaras. Newmarket Press, 1988. Paperback, 106 pages, $5.95.

Here is the best book available for teenagers on the subject of AIDS: factual, readable, and non-judgmental, with clear discussions of how AIDS is transmitted heterosexually, homosexually, or through drug use. Madaras, who writes and lectures widely on the subject of teens and sex, discusses the benefits of abstinence but also includes honest, explicit, but low-key information about safe sex.

MAKING IT: A woman's guide to sex in the age of AIDS, by Cindy Patton and Janis Kelly. Firebrand Books, 1987. Pamphlet, 54 pages, $3.95.

This brief, fully bi-lingual (English-Spanish) guide to AIDS tells how it is spread and how to avoid it. The authors include non-judgmental information for IV-drug users (including directions for cleaning a needle that will be re-used), a section for lesbians and bisexual women, and one about the HIV test. Alison Bechdel's cartoons add a welcome whimsical touch.

MANAGING AIDS IN THE WORKPLACE, by Sam B. Puckett and Alan R. Emery. Addison-Wesley, 1988. Cloth, 191 pages, $19.95.

Most businesses still have not developed policies about how they will respond to AIDS. The time to institute such policies, argue Puckett and Emery, is *before* they are needed. They suggest appropriate policies and workplace programs, and address the legal and ethical considerations that executives must consider.

MORNING-GLORY BABIES: Children with AIDS and the celebration of life, by Tolbert McCarroll. St. Martin's, 1988. Cloth, 161 pages, $14.95.

Here are people who did something about AIDS: A small lay Catholic community opened the doors of its farm home to care for young children born with HIV infections. They overcame the initial hostility of many of its rural neighbors to provide love and a home to children who might otherwise have lived out their lives in a hospital room.

POETS FOR LIFE: Seventy-six poets address AIDS, edited by Michael Klein. Crown, 1989. Cloth, 244 pages, $18.95.

Poetry can express grief, hope, and courage in ways that other writing cannot. Here, seventy-six poets give focus to the deep emotions brought out by the epidemic.

SAFE SEX: The ultimate erotic guide, by John Preston and Glenn Swann. NAL/Plume, 1986. Paperback, 202 pages, $8.95.

For those who are convinced that safe sex can't be much fun, here's a man who thinks otherwise. Former marine Glenn Swann, who does safe-sex shows for gay men, recounts some of his fantasies and experiences in candid detail, showing just how little the requirements of safe sex need cramp one's style.

THE SCREAMING ROOM: A mother's journal of her son's struggle with AIDS, by Barbara Peabody. Avon, 1987. Paperback, 279 pages, $3.95.

This wrenching diary spares nothing as it depicts the author's encounter with AIDS. Others in the same situation may find it helpful to see that they are not alone, but should understand that the book is set in 1984, and while the emotional impact of AIDS has not changed, medical knowledge is much more advanced today.

TEACHING AIDS: A resource guide on acquired immune deficiency syndrome, by Marcia Quackenbush and Pamela Sargent. Network Publications, 1988. Large format paperback, 160 pages, $19.95.

There is widespread agreement that teenagers are not receiving the AIDS education they need, but few teachers have the time to develop teaching materials on their own. This handbook will help tremendously. The authors offer seven curriculum plans covering social studies, health, history, science, and sex education, with worksheets, brief tests, lectures, and background material.

VALLEY OF THE SHADOW, by Christopher Davis. St. Martin's, 1988. Paperback, 208 pages, $7.95.

Of the many novels which now incorporate an AIDS theme, this story of two young men infected by AIDS is easily among the best. Davis is an exceptional writer, and his book poignantly captures the experience that so many people are now confronting.

WHEN SOMEONE YOU KNOW HAS AIDS: A practical guide, by Leonard Martelli, with Fran D. Peltz and William Messina. Crown, 1987. Paperback, 238 pages, $9.95.

Here is practical, intelligent advice for individuals who are providing day-to-day care for a PWA. The book covers emotional, legal, medical, and financial issues that may arise.

Can you use copies of this book in bulk?

Thanks to the generosity of the sponsoring companies, your church, school, business, AIDS agency, or other organization can purchase bulk copies of *You CAN Do Something About AIDS* at a special price of just $50.00 for a box of 100 copies — that works out to only 50 cents a book. Orders must be for multiples of 100 copies, and must be prepaid. Send orders to The Stop AIDS Project, 40 Plympton St., Boston, MA 02118. Include a check or money order for $50 per box of 100 copies, payable to The Stop AIDS Project. Postage is included in the price.

(Sorry, we cannot ship outside the U.S., we cannot invoice you for copies, and we cannot fill orders for less than 100 copies. For smaller quantities, ask your bookseller to stock this title through Ingram Book Company, the country's largest book wholesaler.)

TELEPHONE LISTINGS FOR LOCAL AND STATE ORGANIZATIONS

*Compiled from a longer directory
published by the National AIDS Network*

This listing, compiled with the cooperation of the National AIDS Network, will help you get started if you want to volunteer your time to an AIDS group in your community. This is not a complete listing of AIDS organizations. But the groups listed here can tell you about other organizations in your area. In addition, your local, county, or state health department can often be helpful.

Phone numbers in italics are hotlines offering general information about AIDS, referrals, and sometimes counseling. Other listings are general office numbers.

ALABAMA
  Birmingham: AIDS Outreach, 205-322-0757; 205-322-4197
  Mobile: AIDS Support System, 205-433-6277
  Montgomery: AIDS Outreach, 205-284-2273
ALASKA
  Anchorage: Alaska AIDS Project, 907-276-4880; *800-248-AIDS*
ARIZONA
  Phoenix: Arizona AIDS Project, 602-420-9396
  Tucson: AIDS Project, 602-322-6226; *602-326-AIDS*
ARKANSAS
  Little Rock: Ark. AIDS Foundation, 501-663-7833; *800-448-8305*
CALIFORNIA
  Bakersfield: AIDS Hotline, *800-367-2437*
  Berkeley: Gay Men's Health Collective, 415-644-0425
  Campbell: Aris Project, 408-370-3272
  Concord: Diablo V Community Church, 415-827-2960

Costa Mesa: AIDS Services Foundation, 714-646-0411
Fresno: Central Valley AIDS Team, 209-264-2437
Garden Grove: AIDS Response Program, 714-534-0961
Guerneville: Face to Face, 707-887-1581
Long Beach: Project Ahead, 213-590-9019
Los Angeles: AIDS Project, *213-876-AIDS; 800-922-AIDS*;
   213-962-1600
   Minority AIDS Project, 213-936-4949
Merced: AIDS Support Team, 209-723-5221
Modesto: Stanislaus Community AIDS Project, 209-572-2437
Oakland: AIDS Project of the East Bay, 415-834-8181
Palm Springs: Desert AIDS Project-CCCC, Inc., 619-323-2118
Redding: North State AIDS Project, 916-225-5252
Riverside: Inland AIDS Project, 714-784-2437; *800-451-4133*
Sacramento: AIDS Foundation, 916-448-2437
San Diego: AIDS Project, 619-543-0300; 619-543-0604
San Francisco: AIDS Foundation, 415-864-4376; *800-FOR-AIDS*
   Shanti Project, 415-777-2273
San Luis Obispo: AIDS Task Force, 805-549-5540
Santa Barbara: Tri-Counties AIDS Project, 805-681-5120
Santa Cruz: AIDS Project, 408-427-3900; *408-458-4999*
Santa Rosa: Sonoma County AIDS Project, 707-576-4734;
   707-579-2437
West Hollywood: AIDS Project, 213-876-8951; 213-962-1600
   Shanti Foundation, 213-962-8197

COLORADO
Boulder: Boulder County AIDS Project, 303-444-6121
Denver: Colorado AIDS Project, 303-837-0166

CONNECTICUT
Bantan: N.W. Conn. AIDS Project, 203-482-1596; *203-567-4111*
Hartford: Gay/Lesbian Health Collective, 203-236-4431
New Briton: AIDS Project, *203-225-6789*
New Haven: AIDS Project, 203-624-2437

DISTRICT OF COLUMBIA
Washington: Whitman Walker Clinic/AIDS Program,
   202-332-5295; 202-797-3562

DELAWARE
Wilmington: Delaware Lesbian and Gay Health Advocates
   AIDS Co., 302-652-6776

FLORIDA
Statewide: *800-FLA-AIDS*
Fort Lauderdale: AIDS Center One, 305-485-7175
Key West: AIDS Help, Inc., 305-296-6196

Lakeland: Polk AIDS Support Service, *813-687-AIDS*
Lantana: Comprehensive AIDS Program, 407-845-4400
Miami: Health Crisis Network, 305-326-8833; 800-443-5046;
  305-634-4636
Orlando: Cent. Fla. AIDS Unified Resources Inc., 407-849-1452
Sarasota: AIDS Support, 813-951-1551; *813-951-AIDS*
Tampa: AIDS Network, *813-221-6420*
West Palm Beach: Hospice of West Palm Beach, 407-848-5200

GEORGIA
Athens: AIDS Athens, 404-542-2437
Atlanta: AID Atlanta, 404-872-0600; *800-551-2728*
  Outreach, Inc., 404-873-5992
Macon: Central City AIDS Network, 912-742-2437
Savannah: First City Network, Inc., 912-236-CITY

HAWAII
Honolulu: Life Foundation, 808-971-2437
Kailua: Hawaii Council of Churches, 808-263-9788
Volcano: AIDS Helpline, 808-969-6626

IDAHO
Boise: Idaho AIDS Foundation, 208-345-2277

ILLINOIS
Champaign: Gay Community AIDS Project, 217-351-AIDS
Chicago: AIDS Comprehensive Center, 312-908-9191
  AIDS Foundation, 312-642-5454

INDIANA
Evansville: AIDS Resource Group, 812-423-7791
Fort Wayne: AIDS Task Force, 219-424-0844
Indianapolis: APIC Indiana AIDS Task Force, 317-634-1441;
  317-257-HOPE

IOWA
Des Moines: Cent. Iowa AIDS Project, *800-445-AIDS*
Iowa City: Iowa Center For AIDS/ARC Resources and
  Education, *319-338-2135*
Waterloo: AIDS Coalition of Northeast Iowa, 319-234-6831

KANSAS
Topeka: AIDS Project, 913-232-3100
Wichita: AIDS Referral Services, 316-264-2437

KENTUCKY
Lexington: AIDS Crisis Taskforce, 606-281-5151
Louisville: Comm. Health Trust of Kentucky, 502-636-3341; *502-
454-6699*
Newport: No. Kentucky AIDS Task Force, 606-291-0770

LOUISIANA
Baton Rouge: AIDS Task Force, 504-923-2277
New Orleans: NO/AIDS Task Force, 504-891-3732;
800-992-4379

MAINE
Bangor: Eastern Maine AIDS Network, 207-990-3626
Portland: AIDS Project, 207-774-6877; *207-775-1267*;
800-851-AIDS

MARYLAND
Baltimore: Health Ed. & Resource Org. (HERO), 301-685-1180;
800-638-6252
Rockville: Montgomery County HERO, 301-762-3385

MASSACHUSETTS
Boston: AIDS Action, 617-437-6200; *800-235-2331*
Brighton: Project Win, 617-783-7300
Cambridge: AIDS Family Support Group, 617-491-0600
Worcester: AIDS Project, 508-755-3773

MICHIGAN
Detroit: Michigan AIDS Hotline/AIDS Wellness Networks, 313-547-9040; *800-872-2437*
Wellness House of Michigan, 313-342-1230
Flint: Wellness Networks, Inc., *313-232-0888*
Grand Rapids: AIDS Task Force, 616-459-9177
Hamtramck: Friends, People with AIDS Alliance, 313-543-8310;
800-648-5874
Royal Oak: Health Education Association, Detroit, 313-883-6049
Wellness Networks, 313-547-3783

MINNESOTA
Minneapolis: Minnesota AIDS Project, 612-870-7773;
800-248-AIDS

MISSISSIPPI
Jackson: Mississippi Gay Alliance, 601-353-7611

MISSOURI
Columbia: MID Missouri AIDS Project, 314-875-2437
Kansas City: Good Samaritan Project, 816-561-8784
Free Clinic, 816-231-8896; 816-231-8895
Springfield: AIDS Project/Springfield, 417-864-5594
St. Louis: Effort For AIDS, 314-531-2847; *314-531-7400*

MONTANA
Billings: AIDS Support Network, 406-252-1212

NEBRASKA
Omaha: Nebraska AIDS Project, 402-342-4233; *800-782-AIDS*

NEVADA
Las Vegas: Aid for AIDS of Nevada, 702-369-6162
  Gay Switchboard of Las Vegas, 702-733-9990
Reno: Nevada AIDS Foundation, 702-329-2437
NEW HAMPSHIRE
Manchester: N.H. AIDS Foundation, 603-595-0218
NEW JERSEY
Mahwah: New Jersey Buddies, 201-837-8125
Neptune: AIDS Information Group, 201-758-0077
New Brunswick: AIDS Education Proj., 201-763-0668
  Hyacinth Foundation, 201-246-8439; *800-433-0254*
Newark: N.J. Lesbian & Gay AIDS Awareness, 201-763-2919
  N.J. Lesbian and Gay Alliance/St. Michael's, 201-877-5524
Vineland: Casa Prac, Inc., 609-692-2331
NEW MEXICO
Albuquerque: New Mexico AIDS Services, 505-266-0911
Los Cruces: SW AIDS Committee, 505-525-AIDS
NEW YORK
Albany: AIDS Council, 518-434-4686; *518-445-AIDS*
Bridgehampton: East End Gay Org., 516-324-3699;
  516-385-AIDS
Bronx: Pediatric AIDS Hotline, 212-430-4227; *212-430-3333*
Brooklyn: AIDS Task Force C.S.P., 718-596-4781; *718-638-AIDS*
Buffalo: Western New York AIDS Program, 716-847-2441;
  716-847-AIDS
Dresden: Presbytery of Geneva, 315-536-7753
Huntington Station: Long Island Assoc. for AIDS Care,
  516-385-2451; *516-385-AIDS*
Johnson City: So. Tier AIDS Program, Inc., 607-798-1706;
  607-723-6520; 800-333-0892
New York: Bailey House AIDS Resource Center, 212-206-1001
  Gay Men's Health Crisis, 212-807-6664; *212-807-6655*
  Health Resources Administration, 212-645-7070
Richmond Hill: AIDS Center of Queens County, Inc.,
  718-896-2500
Rochester: AIDS Rochester, Inc., 716-232-3580; *716-232-4430*
Syracuse: AIDS Task Force of Central N.Y., 315-475-2430;
  315-875-AIDS
White Plains: Mid-Hudson Valley AIDS Task Force,
  914-993-0606; *914-993-0607*
NORTH CAROLINA
Asheville: Western N.C. AIDS Project, 704-252-7489
Charlotte: Metrolina AIDS Project, 704-333-1435; *704-333-2437*

Durham: Lesbian & Gay Health Project, 919-683-2182
Greensboro: Triad Health Project, 919-275-1654
Lumberton: Robeson Comm. College Task Force On AIDS,
919-738-7101
Raleigh: AIDS Control Program, 919-733-7301
Wilmington: Grow AIDS Resource Project, 919-675-9222
Winston-Salem: AIDS Task Force, 919-723-5031

OHIO
Akron: AIDS Task Force, 216-375-2960
Canton: AIDS Task Force, 216-489-3231
Cincinnati: Ambrose Clement Health Clinic, 513-352-3139
Cleveland: Health Issues Task Force, 216-621-0766
Columbus: AIDS Task Force, 614-488-2437; 800-332-2437
Painesville: Lake County AIDS Task Force, 216-357-2543
Portsmouth: Southern Ohio AIDS Task Force, *614-353-3339*
Toledo: Area AIDS Task Force, Inc., 419-243-9351
Wapakoneta: Auglaize County AIDS Task Force, 419-738-3410
Youngstown: AIDS Task Force, 216-742-8700

OKLAHOMA
Oklahoma City: Oasis Community Center, 405-525-AIDS
Tulsa: Shanti Tulsa, 918-749-7898

OREGON
Eugene: Willamette AIDS Council, 503-345-7089
AIDS Prevention for Youth, 503-342-2782
Portland: Cascade AIDS Project, 503-223-5907; *800-777-AIDS*
Oregon AIDS Task Force, 503-226-6678

PENNSYLVANIA
Altoona: AIDS Intervention Proj., 814-946-5411; *800-445-6262*
Chester: American Red Cross, 215-874-1484
Harrisburg: So. Central AIDS Assistance Network,
717-238-AIDS
Lancaster: AIDS Project, 717-394-3380; *717-394-9900*
Philadelphia: Action AIDS, 215-981-0088
AIDS Task Force, 215-545-8686; *215-732-AIDS*
Pittsburgh: AIDS Task Force, 412-363-6500; *412-363-2437*;
800-282-AIDS
Reading: Berks AIDS Health Crisis, 215-375-2242
State College: Gay Men's Alliance, 814-237-1950
Upper Darby: Women's Health Concerns, 215-898-8611

RHODE ISLAND
Providence: Project AIDS, 401-831-5522; *800-726-3010*

SOUTH CAROLINA

Columbia: Carolina AIDS Research and Education,
803-777-2273
Palmetto AIDS Life Support Services, 803-779-7257;
800-868-PALS

SOUTH DAKOTA

Sioux Falls: Sioux Empire Gay & Lesbian Coalition,
605-332-4599

TENNESSEE

Chattanooga: Chattanooga Cares, 615-265-2273; 615-757-2745
Knoxville: AIDS Response, *615-523-AIDS*
Memphis: Aid to End AIDS Committee, 901-458-AIDS
AIDS Coalition, 901-726-1690
Nashville: Nashville Cares, 615-385-1510; *615-385-AIDS*

TEXAS

Austin: AIDS Services, 512-472-2273
Corpus Christi: Coastal Bend AIDS Foundation, 512-883-2273;
512-883-5815
Dallas: AIDS Resource Center, 214-521-5124; *214-559-AIDS*
Oak Lawn Counseling Center, 214-520-8108; *214-351-4335*
El Paso: SW AIDS Committee, 915-533-6809; *915-533-5003*
Houston: AIDS Foundation, 713-623-6796; *713-524-2437*
Community AIDS Prevention Project, 713-439-0210
San Antonio: Tavern Guild AIDS Fund, 512-821-6218

VERMONT

Burlington: Vermont Cares, 802-863-2437

VIRGINIA

Charlottesville: AIDS Support Group, 804-979-7714
Headwaters: Elisabeth Kubler-Ross Center, 703-396-3441
Norfolk: Tidewater AIDS Crisis Taskforce, 804-423-5859
Richmond: AIDS Information Network, 804-355-4428;
804-358-AIDS

WASHINGTON

Lacey: Olympia AIDS Task Force, 206-352-2375
Seattle: Northwest AIDS Foundation, 206-329-6923

WISCONSIN

Madison: Madison AIDS Support Network, 608-255-1711
Milwaukee: AIDS Project, 414-273-2437; *800-334-2437*